Introduction to
Daily Yoga Practice

Healthy Living Wellness series

Introduction to Daily Yoga Practice is the first
book in the Healthy Living Wellness series.
The following books represent the complete series:

A Firm Footing in a Changing Marketplace, which
addresses dysfunctional work environments.

Enough is Enough, which addresses
dysfunctional personal financial decisions.

Soy Diversity, which advocates
healthy dietary behavior.

These books can be purchased online
at www.yogaforbusiness.com.

Introduction to Daily Yoga Practice

Bruce Eric Van Horn

ISBN: 0-9724-5122-6

www.yogaforbusiness.com

PHOTOGRAPHY BY TAR
ILLUSTRATIONS BY ROBERT BANDEL
MUSIC BY MICHAEL DIGIROLAMO
BOOK DESIGN AND COMPOSITION BY KELLY & COMPANY, LEE'S SUMMIT, MISSOURI

Contributions

Ten percent of the net royalties from this publication will be directed to the following organizations involved in cancer research and treatment: the Dean and Betty Gallo Cancer Center at the Cancer Institute of New Jersey, and the Gesundheit Institute.

CAUTION: THE AUTHOR AND PUBLISHER RECOMMEND THAT YOU CONSULT WITH YOUR PHYSICIAN BEFORE ENGAGING IN ANY NEW PHYSICAL REGIME, ESPECIALLY IF MEDICAL CONDITIONS ARE PRESENT.

------ ATTENTION: BUSINESSES AND HEALTH CARE ORGANIZATIONS ------

Yoga for Business books are available at quantity discounts with bulk purchase for educational, business, or sales promotional use. For information, please write to: Yoga for Business, 16 Renfrew Road, Chestnut Ridge, N.Y. 10977. Or visit our website at www.yogaforbusiness.com.

Contents

Foreword

There are many paths to enlightenment but they all share common themes because they are effective. I have learned by caring for many people with life threatening illnesses what helps them to save their lives.

Saving one's life isn't about curing an affliction but healing your life and living an authentic life rather than suppressing your feelings and fulfilling the desires of others or trying to impress others.

Bruce's advice is well stated and though it may relate to individual and organizational wellness is basically teaching the same lessons I have seen work for the seriously ill. What is needed besides the information is the inspiration to seek change. I hope the readers will learn what needs to be known now and not wait for a major financial loss or health threat to wake up to the fact that time isn't money. It is everything.

So pay attention to your feelings. Listen to the wisdom of your heart and not just your head. Pay more attention to the things and people you love and who love you. Love is a powerful weapon for healing. Start now and learn how to save your life by eliminating what is killing you.

Bernie Siegel, M.D.
Author *Love, Medicine and Miracles*

Introduction
The Healthy Living Wellness Series

The first six million years of human evolution were no picnic for our ancestors, who usually ended up as lunchmeat for the specialized predators who liked to include them on the menu.

Coming out of the trees was like being cast out of the biblical Garden of Eden. Our ancestors were in a constant state of fear as they were ill equipped for open areas. They became easy prey to the predators that hunted them to near extinction.

Our fight flight response was a means of insuring the survival of our species and communicating danger to others. After a few million years we finally discovered that if we mimicked the behavior of the predators we so feared, we could evolve to become the masters of our world. The organization of human beings into groups was a direct result of the challenges we faced. This fear-based organization was the key to our species success.

Thousands of years ago, the ancient Yogis realized that since we had won the battle over our environment we were finally free to become the masters of ourselves, instead of the prisoners of fear and aggression. However, these teachings were forgotten as man developed more powerful tools to manipulate his environment.

Now fast-forward to the 21st century, and we find that the tools that served us so well in fighting the predators may be contributing

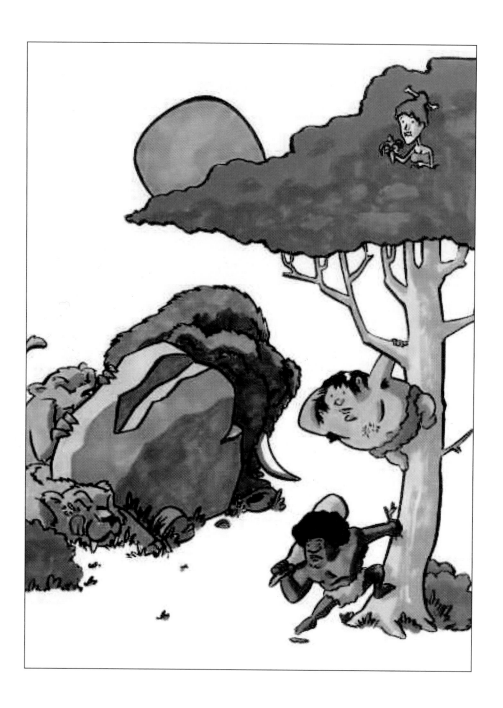

to our health problems and causing global instability. Organizations are still using fear-based motivation as the memory of millions of years of our species struggle haunts our physiology and subconscious mind. These memories and their related behavioral responses can be and have been used to further organizational or nationalistic goals.

Today science and spirituality are on the threshold of a historic re-unification. The tools that were developed thousands of years ago by the ancient wise men hold the key to overcoming our healthcare crises and human suffering. Both Science and Yoga quest for the truth. Science examines observable external forces and Yoga explores the inner realm. Together, these disciplines offer mankind opportunities for furthering our evolutionary process to create a healthier more peaceful world.

The work I have undertaken furthers the work of my Guru the renown Shri Brahmananda Sarasvati, who was known as Ramamurti S. Mishra, M.D. a well respected and loved Yoga Guru and M.D. He dedicated his life to the integration of Eastern and Western sciences, culture and philosophy.

The Guruji suggested that perhaps we have re-entered the garden but have been unaware due to our ignorance. Enlightenment comes when we realize that the majority of our suffering is self-inflicted. We need to move away from predatory-prey patterns of behavior. The key to winning the battle will be in realizing we are the enemy. Make friends with your enemy. Death is not the enemy; ignorance of our mortality is the real villain, which robs us of our life. Be in the moment; be at peace.

The Healthy Living Wellness series presents a number of tools you can use to start to shut down the stress response and aggressive behavior so you can avoid becoming lunchmeat in your personal life and the business world. We all have the capacity to evolve to reach

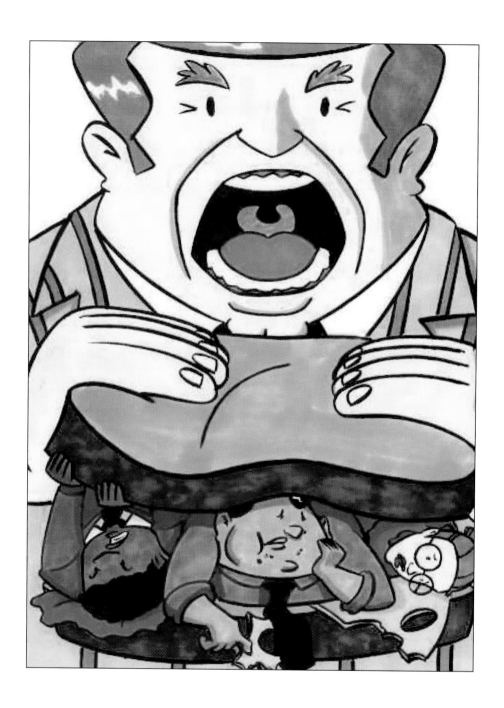

our potential in this lifetime and help the world in its evolution away from fear and aggression. With a positive attitude toward change and growth, you can overcome your doubt and limitations.

The first book, *Daily Yoga Class,* focuses on the specific mind-body exercises that you can use to overcome your fears and realize that you are more than just meat. The second book, *Firm Footing,* explores the way many workplaces continue to make you lunchmeat on a daily basis and tools you can use to protect yourself from predatory behavior. The third book, *Enough is Enough,* shows you how you can place more value on your personal assets as opposed to your things, so the bill collectors don't make you into lunchmeat, and the fourth book, *Soy Diversity,* shows us when we've become meat don't eat, run, that is if you are feeling nervous, anxious or depressed, eating may be the worse thing for you to do. We will present Yogic exercises to burn off that adrenaline and bring you back into balance.

If you can breathe you can do Yoga. Once you gain control over your breathing, you can begin to take control over your body. This program is designed to help you bring your body back into balance gradually, without pain so you can become the master of your inner domain.

Ann Thracks from the Accounting Department, Manny Problemas from Marketing and Oscar Fodder from Operations join us. Our artist has illustrated these characters based on certain archetypal characteristics from Ayurveda, the sister science of Yoga. I use the characters to honor the experiences you have encountered in your lives and to lighten up the subject matter.

We have designed each book to include a four-step program, which includes pet therapy, humor therapy, art therapy, music therapy and experiential learning through Yoga. We are confident that this multi-sensory approach to wellness will help you make positive behavioral changes. While each book stands on its own, it is recommended that you follow the series sequentially to achieve optimal results.

We hope you enjoy the process.

Love

Peace

Bruce Van Horn
CEO Yoga for Business, Inc.

Preface

In our fast-paced environment many people are under tremendous stress. Stress triggers the fight or flight response, in which toxic chemicals are released. Over time this constant stress reaction can compromise the immune system. Practicing Yoga not only can help improve daily performance of activities and enhance creative problem solving but also has the potential to control escalating health care costs.

Yoga is a form of exercise for the body, mind, and spirit. The ancients produced a perfectly bundled, multitasked, and time-efficient practice that can address all our needs, and modern science is beginning to confirm the validity of their philosophical design. By observing nature, such as resting cats and dogs, the ancient sages recognized that certain stretches energized the lymphatic system. A cat can be resting all day, but once it stretches it can jump on top of a refrigerator. The cat isn't concerned about attending an early morning aerobics class. It can tap into its own energy system at any time.

Yoga strengthens the joints without stress, increases lean muscle mass, and enhances flexibility. Yoga can also provide an effective cardiovascular workout as well as improve breathing and metabolization of food and oxygen. Yoga can enhance sexual performance and strengthen orgasm. Yoga has been shown to benefit overall health and functioning of internal organs and tissues.

Yoga also develops discipline and self-confidence. Yoga can help you become a master of yourself instead of a prisoner of your emotions. Yoga can help you become more intuitive, creative, and synchronistic. Finally, if you are a student seeking to find meaning in your life, Yoga can transport you to a state of Dharma, where you understand the purpose of your soul's journey and the true nature of the Universe.

Many people take better care of their cars than they do themselves. Because they are usually devoted to caring for their families and others, they often fail to address their own health issues and in doing so put their families and themselves at risk.

The majority of people I meet are not using all their personal assets in the pursuit of their careers. Often they are using primarily one hemisphere of their brains, relying on only one of their senses, failing to provide the proper resources for their bodies, and rarely if ever engaging in quiet contemplation to find answers from their higher power. If a business were run this way the management would be quickly replaced. As individuals we don't have to fear such a take-over, unless of course we believe in alien abductions. Most of us do, however, want to realize our full potential, as cocreators of the Universe. The technological world we are building will allow us to increase our creative potential.

Leonardo da Vinci is the perfect example of an individual who realized his full potential. In his pursuit of understanding the mysteries of divine creation, he applied Yogic principles hundreds of years ago. When asked about his success he responded this way:

I understand the Art of Science [right-brain thinking].

I understand the Science of Art [left-brain thinking].

I use all my senses when I create.

I understand my purpose in life.

As a CPA and an MBA I have always lectured my clients on how they must maximize the use of their assets to be competitive. In most companies, especially those in the technology sector, the greatest asset is human capital. However, our current financial accounting models ignore this most important element of a business. The result is that we have not devoted adequate resources to our employees, and the valuation of our companies has been distorted. Many large corporations are now beginning to devote resources to preventive health programs, such as in-house Yoga classes. the Healthy Living Wellness series can serve as a catalyst to accelerate and unify this trend.

By combining what I have learned about Yoga and business, I have developed a program that integrates the two and demystifies this ancient Eastern philosophy. As a successful entrepreneur, I have found that the concepts of Yoga and business are congruent. Both are based on an organic interpretation of the organization and the human being as changing and not static. The only certainty is change, and business organizations that understand these principles have the greatest longevity. In my volunteer work as a Yoga instructor working with cancer survivors I have noticed that there is a parallel with individuals: longevity in humans is linked to adaptability to change.

The fear of change is our greatest obstacle because it keeps us locked into rigid patterns of behavior and prevents us from reaching our potential. We fear change because at a very subtle level all our fears are related to our mortality. But we can learn to welcome uncertainty and the unknown as opportunities to pursue our creativity. Yoga is the ideal exercise to reprogram your body and mind toward flexibility and adaptability. Many of the Yogic exercises in this book have been renamed using terms from business, such as Deflating a Bloated Bureaucracy, Bending Over Backward to Serve Your Customers, Firm Footing in a Changing Marketplace, and my favorite, the headstand, which is Change from the Top Down. In addition, some positions have modifications for those with physical limitations.

In Yoga the focus of your mind is as important as the physical position. Yoga is a moving meditation, and each position reflects a state of awareness, a relationship or attitude toward the Universe. Your body is the antenna or receiving channel, and these exercises will open you to creative ideas and solutions to problems.

In order to change and have the freedom to create, businesses typically allocate a percentage of their revenue to research and development. These companies understand that to stay on the cutting edge they have to upgrade their technology. Often individuals don't afford themselves the same opportunity. We get locked into a material lifestyle where we feel a need to compete with our neighbors. This causes us to run faster and faster on the treadmill just to keep up. We do not allocate either the time or the resources for personal growth because we are spending to feed a lifestyle. Many people trade themselves for their self-image, thereby depleting their personal assets.

Our personal assets are body, mind, and spirit. The ultimate goal of Yoga is a union of the three. The meditative state of heightened awareness is the ultimate goal of these exercises. Enlightenment confers many benefits, including finding your purpose (Dharma), understanding your latent talents, experiencing synchronicity, discovering your Karma and how it can be transmuted, and understanding your place as a cocreator of the Universe.

All this talk about spirit might make you a bit uneasy. But please try to suspend your criticism and keep an open mind. Doing so is like hedging a position in the market. You are covering your downside risk. The spiritual exercises and development will at a minimum make you feel more effective in the world, and perhaps they will give you a glimpse of something far grander.

Yoga is not a religion; it is a philosophy and a science. Developed thousands of years ago, it is a systematic approach to wellness and communion with the divine. It seeks to unify and treat all paths and journeys toward enlightenment with respect and admiration. Yoga is cosmic awareness, pure consciousness, which is beyond body, mind, time, and space. It will make your life better.

Currently humankind is looking for clues to our origins in the deep regions of outer space. Science tells us that we are stardust, made of recycled elements that existed as one point of energy at the beginning of the Universe. The intelligence of the Universe flows through every cell of your body, and the answers to the mysteries can be found within.

Through the Healthy Living Wellness series you can more easily achieve your potential, create unlimited wealth, and obtain self-actualization. Come join me for an inner journey to rediscover the self. I am confident that you will enjoy the trip.

Acknowledgments

I would like to offer thanks to gurus of the ages who have inspired me on my journey; they include Moses, Jesus, Lord Shiva, Rumi, the Buddha, Helen Keller, Gandhi, Mother Teresa, Benjamin Franklin, Leonardo da Vinci, Dr. Martin Luther King, Jr., and Albert Einstein. I feel their support and spiritual presence.

To Dr. Bernie Siegel, who taught me to love myself and believe in myself.

I would also like to thank some of my contemporary teachers, such as Andrew Weil, Ram Dass, Bernie Siegel, Deepak Chopra, Patch Adams, and Wayne Dyer.

Further thanks to Bill Jones, Matt Galemmo, and John Lacagnina for the graphics, photography, and production.

To our technical advisors at Odyssey Tech, Richard Delaney, Lou Cortese, Art Aldrich, your contribution and support is deeply appreciated.

Special thanks to the International Association of Yoga Therapists, Sharada, and Debra Dear for their input, and the yogis Bhavani, Beth Lyins, Jill Mahrlig, and Donna Milan.

Behind every great author is a great editor. Jean Lucas, thank you for your patience and good sensibility. Additional gratitude to Chris Angelos for his input.

And special thanks to my illustrator, Robert Bandel; my musician, Michael Di Girolamo; and John Kelly for layout and design.

And finally my Advisory Board members, Bill DeVries, Gregg Spieth, Bill Reisel, Chris Greiner, and many others who have given their time and effort to make this project a reality.

I give thanks to spirit for allowing me to serve.

CHAPTER
ONE
Why Yoga

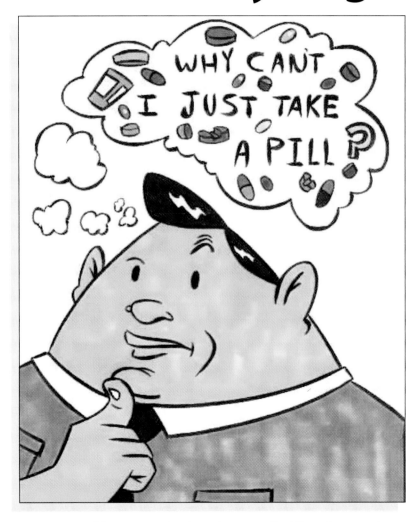

Manny Problemas, Marketing Manager, End Run Corporation

Our country is currently facing yet another health care crisis. Despite the spread of managed care, medical expenses, led by drug prices, continue to surge. This rise has forced many companies to reduce or eliminate health benefits, increasing the percentage of the population that is not covered by insurance. In addition, overall satisfaction with the health care industry is declining, and a larger and larger percentage of the population is critical of managed care. The dissatisfaction has grown so great that it has ignited a movement on Capitol Hill for a patient's bill of rights. But there is little talk of individual responsibility and promoting healthy lifestyle choices.

The pace of the world pushes us at breakneck speeds. Those in fast-track careers in corporate America are often overcome by stress. Even for those not on a fast track, juggling the responsibilities of raising kids when both parents are working can be extremely difficult. As commuting time keeps increasing, we have less and less time for ourselves.

We are constantly being bombarded with all sorts of stimuli, which require our immediate attention. The fight or flight response is often triggered, and a chemical change ensues that affects every cell in our bodies. The continuous release of the hormone adrenaline can wreak havoc on a body.

Both in the workplace and at home, we are often overwhelmed, and our immune systems respond in ways that lead to lack of energy, grumpiness, increased absenteeism, chronic illness, work-related injuries, and turnover. These effects not only harm the bottom line of the company but the well-being and quality of life of the family.

Numerous studies have identified the following factors as causing the most stress in men and women:

1. Death of a spouse or family member
2. Divorce, separation, or marital conflicts

The Effects of Stress in the United States of America

Stress is America's number-one health problem, costing the U.S. economy $300 billion annually.

43 percent of all adults suffer health problems caused by stress.

75 to 90 percent of all visits to primary care physicians are for stress-related complaints or disorders.

Stress is responsible for more than half of the 550 million workdays lost to absenteeism annually.

A three-year study by a large corporation showed that more than 60 percent of employee absences were caused by psychological problems such as stress.

Workers' compensation costs for stress-related illnesses have skyrocketed and threaten to bankrupt the system. In California alone the costs from such claims now exceed $1 billion annually. Nine out of ten job-stress lawsuits are successful, with an average payout of more than four times that of regular injury claims.

40 percent of all worker turnover is the result of job stress.

Workplace violence is rampant. Homicide is the second leading cause of fatal occupational injury and the leading cause of death for working women.

Immune disturbances from the common cold and herpes to arthritis and AIDS have been linked to stress. Recent research has confirmed the important role stress plays in causing cardiovascular disease, cancer, gastrointestinal disorders, skin conditions, and neurological and emotional disorders.

The market for stress management programs, products, and services amounted to over $10 billion in the year 2000.

3. Injury or health issues for self or family member

4. Balancing work and family responsibilities

5. Workplace issues such as termination, performance reviews, etc.

6. Retirement

7. Sexual difficulties

8. Moving

The Healthy Living Wellness series provides you with tools you can use daily to better cope with stressful events so that you can maintain your health and the health of your family. You will enhance your own self-understanding, thereby setting the tone for harmonious, loving relationships. And you will improve your ability to adapt to change and cope with special needs or challenges.

The Healthy Living Wellness series is beneficial in the workplace as well. By relearning that authority and power are equated with productivity, integrity, and creativity, employees will feel empowered and willing to embrace the organization's goals. As a result, customer relationships will improve and the organization will prosper.

In many cases it's not individuals' lack of education or technical training that hinders the growth of a company but their approach to dealing with customers and employees. Yoga and meditation can change the way we interact with others, not only at work but also at home. All will welcome the daily benefits from these improved relationships.

Industries may come and go, as may businesses, but if we stay flexible we can re-create ourselves daily and develop the goods and services demanded by the marketplace. We need to learn not to fear change but to embrace it. By letting go of the fear we can become more effective in addressing the needs of our clients and customers and in motivating our employees to share our vision of the future. When we focus on giving, our family relationships will improve and our sex lives will be enhanced.

The Healthy Living Wellness series can help transport you to a more calming and comforting reality. All you need is an open mind and the desire to make minor changes in your life. Your body is in a constant state of change. At the cellular level you are re-creating yourself every few months. Yoga can make you more flexible and adaptable to changes in your life and in the world around you.

Back in the '80s I was pursuing a fast-track career in corporate America; when I came down with an ulcer that almost put me in the hospital, I knew I had to start making some life changes. Perhaps like many of you I had always associated Yoga with left-wing refugees from the sixties. I believed it was an escape from reality. But I found that Yoga connects us to the present by quieting the mind's thoughts about the past and the future. I found it difficult at first to train my mind to stop thinking about the past and the future. In a world focused on the bottom line, we become biased toward observable, tangible action. Practicing Yoga can help you overcome the bias of your senses and social conditioning at work and at home. People can learn to practice Yoga and meditation to improve the quality of their lives.

The daily practice of Yoga can help you become more productive in your career and more peaceful in your personal life. Ultimately Yoga can help you enjoy your life fully. What form of physical exercise does all this? What physical activity can you do anywhere, any time, without any investment in equipment? It's like having your shrink, place of worship, and health club all rolled into one—the perfect combination for any man or woman.

The wide range of benefits from practicing Yoga are noted in Table 1.1, which was prepared by the International Association of

Yoga Therapists. For each physiological change associated with Yoga it lists corresponding psychological and biochemical changes.

My first Yoga class was an accident. A friend invited me to her exercise class. When I arrived I realized it was Yoga, and I was the only male. It had already started when we got there, so it was too late for me to leave. I figured I would just go along with it, and go to the gym for a real man's workout later that afternoon. But in five minutes I was sweating and panting on the floor, while the others in the class glided gracefully from one pose to another. How could this be? I realized that Yoga wasn't for sissies.

I had tried many other forms of exercise, but I never achieved my fitness goals because I was not breathing correctly. Yoga taught me how to breathe, and then I was able to achieve my physical potential. I may not be Arnold Schwarzenegger, but I have a better body now than when I was sixteen.

Table 1.2, also prepared by the International Association of Yoga Therapists, compares the benefits of Yoga and traditional exercise.

Some people have the mistaken notions that Yoga is painful and that Yogis are just masochists in turbans. I too had these preconceptions, but I soon realized that pain was a judgment I was placing on a feeling I was unaccustomed to. When I stopped judging that feeling as painful I began to excel. Now I think of it as surrender. When you reach advanced levels of Yoga you can stretch yourself into positions where you can finally surrender to something greater than yourself, and it feels great. In a way it's similar to orgasm. Do you consider the tension that precedes an orgasm painful? If you succumb to the feeling you judge as painful, you will never experience the bliss of inner peace that Yoga can provide.

This book offers an introduction to various Yogic exercises, which you can use as the basis for your daily Yoga practice. It will take you

TABLE 1.1 Benefits of Yoga

Physiological Benefits	Psychological Benefits	Biochemical Effects
Autonomic nervous system equilibrium stabilizes, with a tendency toward parasympathetic nervous system dominance rather than the usual stress-induced sympathetic nervous system dominance	Somatic and kinesthetic awareness increase	Glucose decreases
Pulse rate decreases	Mood improves and subjective well-being increases	Sodium decreases
Respiratory rate decreases	Self-acceptance and self-actualization increase	Total cholesterol decreases
Blood pressure decreases (of special significance for hyporeactors)	Social adjustment increases	Triglycerides decrease
Galvanic skin response increases	Anxiety and depression decrease	HDL cholesterol increases
Alpha brain waves increase (theta, delta, and beta waves also increase during various stages of meditation)	Hostility decreases	LDL cholesterol decreases
EMG activity decreases	Psychomotor functions improve	VLDL cholesterol decreases
Cardiovascular efficiency increases	Grip strength increases	Cholinesterase increases
Respiratory efficiency increases (respiratory amplitude and smoothness increase, tidal volume increases, vital capacity increases, breath-holding time increases)	Dexterity and fine motor skills improve	Catecholamines decrease

(continued on next page)

TABLE 1.1 *(continued)*

Physiological Benefits	Psychological Benefits	Biochemical Effects
Gastrointestinal function normalizes	Eye-hand coordination improves	ATPase increases
Endocrine function normalizes	Choice reaction time improves	Hematocrit increases
Excretory functions improve	Steadiness improves	Hemoglobin increases
Musculoskeletal flexibility and joint range of motion increase	Depth perception improves	Lymphocyte count increases
Posture improves	Balance improves	Total white blood-cell count decreases
Strength and resiliency increase	Integrated functioning of body parts improves	Thyroxine increases
Endurance increases	Cognitive function improves	Vitamin C increases
Energy level increases	Attention improves	Total serum protein increases
Weight normalizes	Concentration improves	
Sleep improves	Memory improves	
Immunity increases	Learning efficiency improves	
Pain decreases	Symbol coding improves, depth perception improves, flicker fusion frequency improves	

TABLE 1.2   The Advantages of Yoga Compared to Traditional Exercise

Yoga	Traditional Exercise
Parasympathetic nervous system (relaxation response) dominates	Sympathetic nervous system (fight or flight response) dominates
Subcortical regions of the brain are used (associated with well-being); Yoga can help reverse or eliminate addictive behavior	Cortical regions of the brain are used (associated with primary functions)
Slow, dynamic movements	Rapid, forceful movements
Normalization of muscle tone	Increased muscle tension
Low risk of injuring muscles and ligaments	Higher risk of injuring muscles and ligaments
Low caloric consumption	Moderate to high caloric consumption
Effort minimized	Effort maximized
Energizing (breathing is kept natural or controlled)	Fatiguing (breathing is taxed)
Balanced activity of opposing muscle groups	Imbalanced activity of opposing muscle groups
Noncompetitive, process-oriented	Competitive, goal-oriented
Internal awareness	External awareness
Limitless possibilities for growth in self-awareness	Boredom factor

Reprinted with Permission of IAYT. Copyright 1999 by Trish Lamb Feurstein.

through each pose and give you specific instructions on positioning your body and focusing your mind. You should find using this book enjoyable and humorous. Various positions have been renamed and customs modified so you can enjoy the learning process. Chapter 7 offers a meditation I developed to help you incorporate positive changes into your life. The enclosed CD is designed to aid you during your regular Yoga practice. It's recommended that you read this book the first time through and then use the CD in following Yoga workouts.

The photographs show an advanced practitioner to give you an appreciation of your potential. In addition there are instructions for Yoga positions that can be performed in the workplace and modified positions for beginners and those with physical limitations. The Yoga practices in this book are somewhat eclectic and draw upon the ancient traditions of Hatha, including Ananda, Sivananda, and Tantra, of which Kundalini is a part.

I invite you to join me on this journey of self-discovery and personal improvement. With persistence and hard work you can achieve your peak physical condition, improve your performance on the job, and possibly better understand the purpose of your life. Is our souls' journey merely to accumulate material possessions, or is there a deeper meaning? Ultimately the goal of Yoga is to integrate your practice into daily living so that each step you make, each breath you take is done with mindfulness. In this way your life becomes a meditation in action and fundamental enlightenment is possible.

I hope to inspire you with my words and encourage you to proceed.

As you begin this journey I offer you this Hebrew blessing: "May you walk with the spirit, the light of the divine, for all of the days of your life."

Love

Peace

Namaste
(The spirit in me
honors the spirit in you.)

CHAPTER

TWO

Four Step Program for Individual and Organizational Wellness

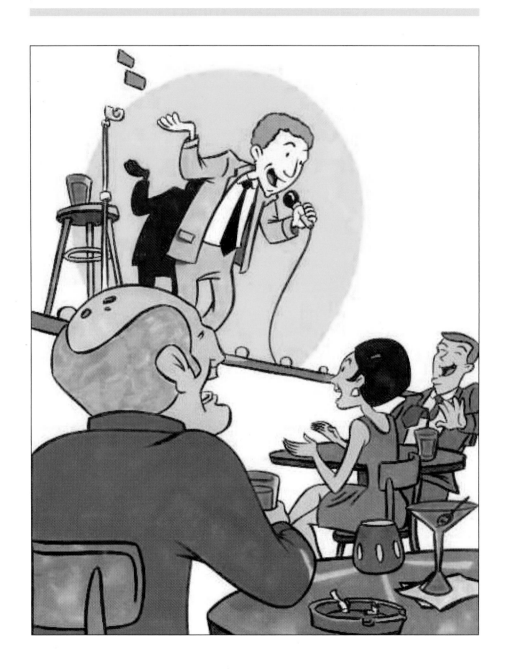

Step One: Discovering the Inner Comic

I feel pretty good . . . But I used to feel like a shleppy Jewish accountant when I would get the 6:30 train to come into the "City" to do your taxes. . . .

My life got really interesting when I married this Greek Orthodox Mormon Cosmetic Opera Singer from Utah . . . God if my life were a movie it might be called the Night Jerry Seinfeld met the New Age Marie Osmond at Zorba's Alcohol Free Restaurant. Not only do I have a demanding Jewish mother with a split personality, but an ex-wife who has put a contract out on my life, and five mother-in-laws from the polygamist state of Utah that hate Jews and like to throw plates. So to piss them all off I quit my Jewish job as an accountant and became a Yoga instructor working with men who have erectile dysfunctions. Now they're all confused.

But the worst thing is, when I get into a fight with my wife the mother-in-laws start running personal ads in the *Salt Lake City Tribune* that read something like this.

> Oppressed Mormon Woman with a Biological Clock Deadline Seeks Mormon Knight to Rescue Her From Her Cheap Jew Husband Who Won't Give Her Any Kids

I remember how jealous my parents were as a child growing up when they would learn that their friends were getting a divorce. . . . The Weinbergs are getting divorced . . . they're happy . . . they have money . . . we're poor so we got to stay together and be miserable till death do us part.

You know, my father also used to talk about suicide. He would say that he wished he had a garage so that he could go out in style.

So when I grew up I chose a career where I could afford a divorce and an assisted suicide and I got this huge two-car garage that Dr.

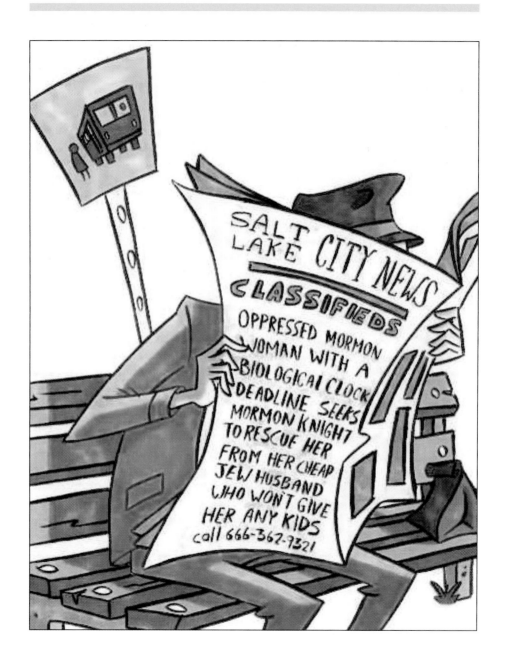

Kervorkian helped me renovate so when my kids get ready to ship me off to the home . . . and you know they will because my Jewish American Princesses aren't going to change my Depends . . . I can get the last laugh.

You know humor is a great way to heal the pain we have experienced in our lives. With humor, I am trying to transform my pain into a more meaningful experience like: A spot on the Leno show, a house in Beverly Hills, and vacations at the Betty Ford Clinic.

So the Raja Rama, a character I created for healing says, *"uncover the pain, honor it, laugh out loud, and get on with your life."*

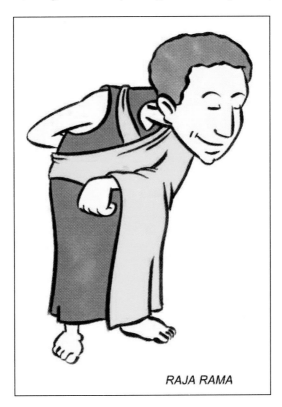

RAJA RAMA

MORAL OF THE STORY

We can't live life without experiencing some form of pain; it is part of the human experience. Pain gives meaning to our life's journey and can lead us back to the path of growth and the pursuit of our life's purpose. Humor can help us to honor the pain and acknowledge it. Unfortunately most of us repress our pain and emotions, anesthetizing ourselves with addictions such as alcohol, drugs, food, nicotine, sex, money, material possessions, work, relationships, etc. In my own life I went through a series of addictions. You name the addiction . . . I had it. In fact, if it weren't for me, my therapist wouldn't have been able to send his children to Ivy League schools.

Many psychiatrists, psychologists, and pharmaceutical companies think we should all be taking daily doses of Prozac; but again, this is just another addiction causing the power to be taken from you. What we really need is to get in touch with our true feelings, which is what the addiction is preventing us from doing in the first place. Yoga practice allows us to evaluate our emotions and feelings from a balanced, objective place. Overcoming our addictions is one of the spiritual lessons we come to experience in this life. Will we have the courage to admit that we have these addictions, and will we have the courage to take the action necessary?

Many of us never get the courage to face our addictions and we continue to blame others for our failings. This pattern of behavior was taught to us in early childhood. We learned by fear that if we placed the blame on others we could escape punishment.

I recall a time when I was five years old. I had colored the solar system on the living room wall in crayon. When my mother asked me who did it, I told her that it was my one-year-old sister. When my mother began to praise my sister's genius, I quickly admitted that it was my creation. I was given a bucket and a sponge and I remember scrubbing all day long.

Many parents are quick to react to such behavior with a physical and verbal assault. This conditions the child to avoid accepting responsibility. The results are that we have organizations full of individuals who have been socialized to lie and blame others for their shortcomings and who fail to stand up for their beliefs. Our legal, healthcare, and educational systems have further contributed to removing the burden of personal responsibility to the detriment of the individual and society as a whole.

I have found that many people facing life-challenging illnesses are willing to accept responsibility for their actions and dispense with the denial process because it is obviously no longer serving their best interests. In working as a Yoga therapist with cancer patients I have found it very important to begin to unlock the energy blockages in the body because all of our experiences get manifested in our physiology. Therefore I consider the use of humor to be the first step in healing and healthy living. So as a first exercise construct your own comedy act. You may want to take a few painful experiences from your life and exaggerate them. Humor is often about creating absurdity out of the stuff of everyday life. Sometimes our lives are absurd. In these cases you will not have to be as creative. I have provided about half a page for your act. Please fill in your name. I suggest you may want to share your act with a friend or co-worker. Sharing can be especially healing because it allows us to better understand each other's challenges and past journey. However, do not feel obligated to share. We also will be running a contest for the best Inner Comic. Please submit your submissions to www.yogafor-business.com.

_____'s Comedy Act:

You know if my life were a movie it would be called:

_____

(visit the www.fandango.com site under Hot Movies and choose from a genre. Your life may fall into one of these categories; Action, Comedy, Drama, Suspense, Romance, Family, Sci-fi or Art House. Once you have chosen your category you can search through an alphabetical listing of movies in your category to find the one that best fits your life.)

(Go ahead and complain like my Jewish grandmother) Not only do I have a _____, but a _____, and a _____, and a _____.

Now write your story. Exaggerate and be absurd with your own faults as well as others in your life. _____

_____

_____

_____

_____

_____

_____

Now see if you can touch upon the more painful experiences with humor _____

_____

_____

_____

_____

_____

_____

_____

_____

End by telling what the sequel to your movie will be called:

_____

Step Two: Discovering the Inner Artist

In the Yoga section, our talented artist, Robert Bandel, has illustrated three characters I have created; Annie, Manny, and Oscar, based on certain archetype characteristics. The characters perform the Yoga positions along with photographs of myself. I use the characters to honor the difficulties you may encounter as well as to lighten up the subject matter. This should be fun and lighthearted, not heavy and painful. The characters allow us to explore some of our traits and behaviors that are similar and possibly uncover some of the limitations we impose on ourselves.

Expressing ourselves through art has also been part of the human experience for tens of thousands of years.

With the assistance of our talented artist, I have created a few illustrations of what I believe were some of the more painful experiences from my life.

On the right sidebar I would like you to honor your experience by creating an illustration. Please try not to be judgmental of your artistic ability, just focus on re-creating the painful experience and adding an absurdity to create some space between you and the experience.

Once the pain has been uncovered, the more difficult process of forgiveness can begin. Through Yoga and exercises in detachment you

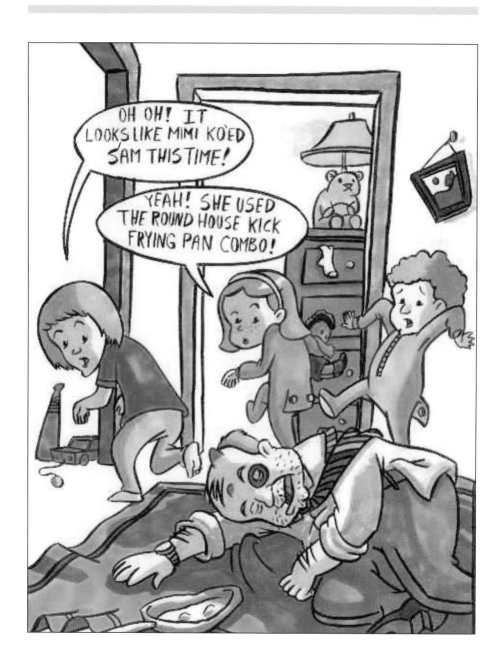

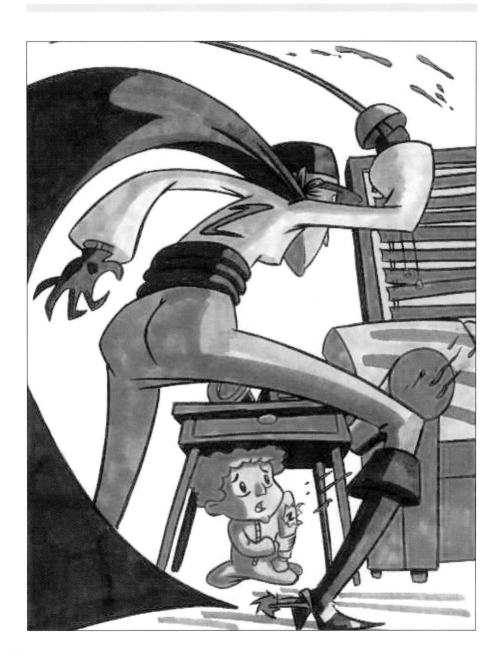

can start to experience your life from a place of greater understanding and tolerance. In this way you can create the space to begin to understand the challenges and limitations of those who may have hurt you in the past. You may also be able to begin looking at how you may be contributing to the melodrama in your life and how you can avoid it in the future. We will explore some techniques for accomplishing this later in the book.

Step Three: Discovering Your Inner Musician

There is an underlying vibration throughout the Universe that dates back to the original "Big Bang" some 8 to 12 billion years ago. There is also a vibration that runs through our physiology that is related to our heartbeat and breathing. Even our thoughts have a sound associated with them. Therefore, everything has its own theme music, no matter how silent it appears.

When our thoughts are out of kilter, they throw off our normally relaxed patterns of breathing, and heartbeat.

Our talented musician, Michael DiGirolamo, has created a musical combination for the meditations in the accompanying CD that will help you move from patterns of thought that tend to disrupt the system, to patterns of thought that lead to relaxation, focus, and healing. The music for the Yoga practice has been coordinated with the movement to open energy patterns in the areas of the body being stretched.

As an exercise in breathing and in vibration awareness, I suggest you purchase a basic C chord harmonica. The harmonica is a great instrument because we can make sounds both on the inhalation and exhalation. What I suggest is that you work toward a four-second inhalation and a six-second exhalation. This is a very healing interval.

By getting six breaths per minute you are training your entire physiology to slow down and assume a healthier beat and rhythm.

To make the exercise even more interesting, you can vary your position on the harmonica, using higher notes and lower notes. You can even shake the harmonica in your mouth to create interesting sounds.

I recommend practicing the musical exercise at least five minutes a day until you feel comfortable with breathing intervals. Or feel free to continue to use the harmonica. It is a wonderful instrument, which I have found to be very healing.

Step Four: Loving Your Self

While it is true that as human beings we all need to experience some pain on our journey, there comes a point in time when we no longer need to inflict suffering upon ourselves. Self-love involves understanding that you are complete and whole and not lacking in any regard. You are a microcosm of the Universe. A hologram of creation is inside each of us. We all have great power, but we have been afraid to uncover it. The uncovering takes great courage because what I am asking you to do is to step into the silence. This involves tuning out the problems of the world we ultimately wish to solve. Only by creating this distance can you be effective.

In music the silence gives the notes meaning. In your life the silence can do the same. To be effective you must make a commitment now to yourself and your well being to immerse yourself fully in this program. Allocate the time required, which is about an hour each day. I suggest you try the program for a month. I am confident that once you experience the positive changes, you will make it a lifelong pursuit and wonder how you ever survived without it.

There are many forces that don't want you to uncover your inner power because it will mean they lose power over you. Some of the greatest offenders are family members, organized religion, the health-care industry, business organizations, the media, and the government. Unlocking your personal power is one of the great gifts of Yoga practice.

Yoga practice requires discipline, and time. It is so much easier to embark on this path when we have the time and our health is good. Yet we often do not, and wait for a crisis or breakdown before we take action. The key to developing the discipline is to practice self-love. You have to love yourself enough to give yourself this time.

So let's talk more about Yoga and how we can unlock some of the blockages in the body with physical postures and meditation.

CHAPTER THREE

Tips for Beginning Yoga Practice

Before beginning your Yoga practice, you'll need to consider some practical details.

When to Practice

It is helpful to practice once a day. Practicing first thing in the morning is best because it helps prepare you for the day. Also, if you put your practice off until later in the day, you may never get to it. And it is best to practice on an empty stomach. Before dinner is also a good time as long as you don't get distracted.

Where to Practice

You should practice in a quiet place where you will not be disturbed. If you attend a Yoga class, remember that Yoga is about going within and not about competition. Be forgiving of the condition of your body and take pride in your gradual accomplishments.

How Long to Practice

The Yoga program in this book should take about an hour for the exercises and fifteen minutes for the meditation. You can extend or condense the time depending on how long you hold your positions. Beginners may want to start out with 15-second intervals on and off. I have built up to about 60 seconds in each pose. Remember that you should always continue breathing in each position.

What to Wear

Comfortable, loose-fitting clothing is a must. A few blankets are also helpful because as you go into deep states of meditation your body temperature will lower as a result of your metabolic processes slowing down. In addition, I recommend a thick rubber mat, which can be purchased at a sporting goods store. Your Yoga instructor may have extension straps to help you reach certain positions or you can purchase these as well. Practice Yoga in your stocking feet or bare feet.

What to Look At

In general, try to keep your eyes shut except when in standing or balancing positions. Imagine an Olympic high diver before he jumps: His eyes are open, but he is not focused on anything in particular. He has gone within.

What to Focus Your Mind On

When you start your Yoga practice you will be primarily focused on what to do with your body. As your practice develops the positions will feel more natural and you will begin to gain control over your awareness. The Healthy Living Wellness series includes a series of positive affirmations, which can be your focus as you hold your positions. Eventually you may let go of these as well and just focus on the breathing or a mantra. A mantra is a repeated phrase that, like a boat, guides you past your thoughts into the meditative state. Mantras will be discussed in more detail in Chapter 8.

What to Eat

FOOD

There is an inherent intelligence in food. In our attempt to improve efficiency in food production we have sacrificed quality for quantity. The law of cause and effect is clearly demonstrated by our food industry. Perhaps it is not just red wine that gives Europeans better health but their lifestyle and relationship to food. The fast-food mentality is harmful to our collective health. If we look to the animal kingdom for guidance, we notice that there is no incidence of osteoporosis because animals follow their natural instincts. If we can get in touch with our natural instincts, then many diseases, which are really the results of lifestyle choices, can be avoided.

The wisdom of our physiology has provided us with six tastes:

Sweet: Pasta, bread, wheat, grains, meat, fish, seafood, fruits

Sour: Milk, yogurt, lemon, vinegar, and all salad dressings

Salt: Self-explanatory

Bitter: Green leafy vegetables, such as spinach

Astringent: Beans, lentils, tofu

Pungent: Spices, mustard

Ayurveda, the science of life, developed in conjunction with Yoga, the science of union with the divine. Ayurvedic nutrition recommends that we have at least one meal a day that includes all six tastes. The reason we have so many problems with obesity and health is that the typical American diet is out of balance. It is primarily sweet, sour, and salt: French fries and ketchup. When we utilize all the tastes that nature has provided us, we can come back into balance. In addition to more fruit and vegetables we need to add new food groups, like soy and legumes, to our diets.

Reducing consumption of meat will lower testosterone levels, aiding in the fight against prostate cancer. In addition, studies have shown that meat consumption increases aggressiveness. For maximum benefits to your Yoga practice and meditation I recommend reducing meat consumption and substituting fish, especially fatty fish such as salmon, and soy products.

For those with prostate cancer the following foods and or nutrients may be helpful:

Tomatoes

Zinc and vitamin B6

Saw palmetto (160 to 320 milligrams per day)

Amino acids: glycine, alanine, and glutamic acid

Bee pollen

Pax ginseng

PC-SPES (herbal mixture of baikal, skullcap, rabdosia, mum, dyer's woad, Chinese licorice, reishi, and saw palmetto)

Please consult with your physician before starting to take supplements.

FASTING

Fasting may also be useful in helping you to change your eating habits permanently and for cleansing toxicity built up over a lifetime. I recommend fasting only if you have the guidance of a teacher and you coordinate your fasting with your doctor. A fast may enhance your appreciation of eating and all the wonderful natural foods that are available to you.

It is most important to eat as slowly as possible and to be present in the moment when you are eating. Being aware will help you avoid eating to satisfy emotions. Properly chewing your food and pacing yourself will help you avoid many stomach problems and weight management issues. These benefits will ultimately improve your Yoga practice.

Dry Body Brush

Starting your day with a two-minute full body and scalp massage with a natural fiber brush will improve circulation and can reduce hair loss. You can purchase such a brush at your local health food store. Start with the scalp and work down over the back, then chest, arms, buttocks and pelvis, legs, and feet.

Attitude

Your journey can be successful only if you approach Yoga practice with an open mind. You will need to suspend judgment, criticism, doubt, perfectionism, and competition, and replace such negative thoughts with acceptance, compassion, and dogged persistence. You will need to listen to your body and not attempt to push yourself before you are ready. There should be gain without pain.

Do not feed your mind images and thoughts that will agitate it. You may want to avoid the melodrama of the daily news or images of violence and distress. This doesn't mean that you should be aloof from suffering, but you can deal with it more effectively from a place of detachment.

CHAPTER
FOUR
The Body

Yoga practice consists of breathing exercises (pranayama) and Yoga postures (asanas). We will first explore the various breathing exercises and correct sitting positions. The benefits of each pose will be discussed.

Chakras

The word *chakra* is Sanskrit for "wheel" or "disk" and signifies one of the seven basic psychoenergetic centers of the body through which *Prana* or life energy circulates. There are colors associated with the chakras, as described below. Yoga helps to open the energy channels in the body and release any blocks in chakra regions. The most important energy channel runs from the base of the spine to the crown of the head.

Chakra One: Located at the base of the spine and related to physical identity and the basic survival instinct; associated with red, symbolizing health, security, and material prosperity

Chakra Two: Located in the abdomen and related to emotions and the sexual organs; associated with orange, symbolizing adaptability

Chakra Three: Located in the solar plexus and related to one's energy center and personal power; associated with yellow, symbolizing effectiveness

Chakra Four: Located in the heart region and related to love; associated with green, symbolizing self-acceptance and love

Chakra Five: Located in the throat and related to creativity and communication; associated with blue, symbolizing self-expression

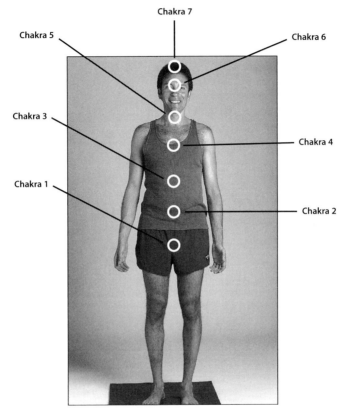

FIGURE 4.1 *The energy chakras*

Chakra Six: Located between the eyebrows and related to self-reflection, inner light, and wisdom; associated with indigo, symbolizing intuition

Chakra Seven: Located at the crown and related to higher states of consciousness; associated with white and violet, symbolizing wisdom

Forgiveness

I have found that forgiveness is the most powerful tool we have for healing. When you can forgive others you empower yourself and you aid in your healing. I recommend that when you reach your point of resistance in these exercises, focus on sending forgiveness to yourself and others and feel the blockages beginning to open.

Breathing

Before you begin it is important to understand the role of breathing in your Yoga practice. *Prana,* the ancient Sanskrit term for "breath," also means "life." This is because the intelligence of the Universe travels effortlessly through your physiology with every breath. The breath is a vessel that can help transport you to a calmer, more focused reality. You will notice a direct relationship between the breath and each Yogic position. The inhalation or exhalation that should accompany each movement of a position will be indicated in its description.

In some cases, as when you go into deep states of meditation, your breathing will be very gentle. At other times, as in certain Kundalini positions, your breathing will be very rapid and deep.

Most people breathe from the chest. When we get stressed we tend to hold on to our breath and tighten our abdominal muscles. For Yoga you want to relax and loosen those abdominal muscles. We will practice some deep Yoga breathing to help with this release. All breathing should arise from deep in your belly and should come through your nose to slow down your breath and stimulate the third chakra, associated with energy.

Try this simple exercise. Sit comfortably in a chair, close your eyes, and imagine you are snorkeling on a tropical coral reef. Place one hand on your abdomen and notice how your breath flows in a long, natural, rhythmic motion corresponding to the ebb and flow of the tide. Now take some long, deep breaths in through your nose and then gently exhale through your nose. Try this breathing pattern for 60 seconds or approximately six rounds. Afterward sit with your eyes closed and notice the changing energy patterns. You may experience a calming sensation and enhanced attentiveness and clarity. Perhaps not much of anything has happened, but with continuing practice the benefits will become more apparent.

Here are the benefits of Yogic breathing:

1. Reduces tension and anxiety

2. Strengthens the immune system

3. Increases metabolism

4. Keeps lung tissue elastic, allowing you to take in more oxygen

5. Tones the abdominal area

6. Improves posture

In Yoga your body moves in four directions: forward, backward, sideways, and twisting. You should exhale at the beginning of each position except the back bends, which commence with an inhalation. As you practice, the breathing will gradually occur naturally.

Movement

All movements in Yoga should be slow and graceful. Hatha Yoga is really a moving meditation in which each position represents a different attitude toward the Universe. You are an antenna to the cosmic mind. By slowing down your movements you can more easily attain the meditative state in a position, thereby increasing the depth and intensity of the seated meditation to follow. In addition, you can reduce the risk of injury, gain better control of your breathing, and enable more muscles to share in the workload, thereby improving conditioning.

Remember that it is better to bend your legs and arms in any given position than to risk injury. Over time you can gradually challenge yourself to straighten out in a pose.

Generally each pose will include first bending in one direction and then bending in the opposite direction.

The first postures you'll need to master in order to begin your Yoga practice are the seated postures.

Seated Postures

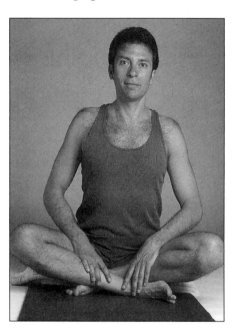

FIGURE 4.2

The primary position for meditation and many Kundalini breathing exercises is a seated posture. Many Westerners will find that their knees are a few inches higher than their hips when they sit cross-legged on the floor. I recommend that you use a pillow or thickly folded blanket to elevate your buttocks to the point where your knees drop to at least the level of your hips. Make sure that you are not sitting against a wall but your spine is straight. (See Figure 4.2.)

If you find that cross-legged sitting is too painful, you can position yourself against a wall for support. When your legs get tired, you can extend them in front of you. Gradually you can build flexibility so you can sit through Yoga positions and meditation.

For those with physical limitations, a chair sitting posture is perfectly acceptable. (See Figure 4.3.)

1. Use a sturdy, armless chair and sit near the front edge of the seat without leaning against the back. If your legs are not perpendicular with the floor, put a phone book either under your feet or under your buttocks.

2. Rest your hands in your lap with your palms facing up.

3. Lift your chest and balance your head over your torso so you can feel the alignment in your spine.

EASY POSTURE

The recommended seated posture for beginners is the Easy Posture. This is a steady and easy position for both Kundalini breathing exercises and meditation. (See Figure 4.2.)

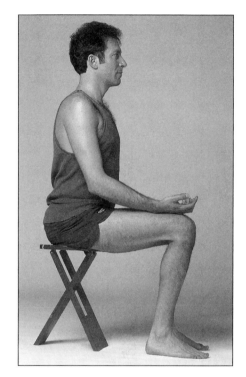

FIGURE 4.3

1. Sit on the floor with your legs out in front of you.

2. Cross your legs at the ankles, with the right leg on top of the left.

3. Place your palms on your knees and push in so that your right foot is underneath your left knee and your left foot underneath your right knee.

4. Lift your chest and balance your head over your torso so you can feel the alignment in your spine.

All the work is being done from your lower belly; your diaphragm should be soft.

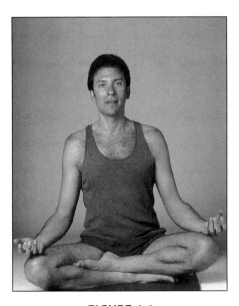

FIGURE 4.4

PERFECT POSTURE (LOTUS POSITION)

A more advanced posture is sometimes referred to as the Lotus Position or the Perfect Posture. This posture is very helpful for men with prostate problems because it opens the first and second chakra regions. The Perfect Posture also improves flexibility in the ankles, knees, and especially the hips. In addition, it will strengthen the back and help deepen the meditative state of awareness. (See Figure 4.4.)

1. Sit on the floor with your legs out in front of you, arms to the sides, and shake out your legs to loosen the muscles.

2. Bend your right knee and bring the heel into the groin, near the perineum. Stabilize your right ankle with your left hand.

3. Bend your left knee and slide your left heel toward the front of your right ankle.

4. Lift your left foot. Position your left ankle just above your right ankle and bring your left heel into the groin area.

5. Tuck the outside of your left foot between your right thigh and calf.

6. Gently place your hands on your knees with palms facing up.

7. Lift your chest and balance your head over your torso so you can feel the alignment in your spine.

Inversions

An inversion is a position in which the normal upright position of the body is reversed, as in the headstand, handstand, or shoulder stand. Inversions are the most powerful Yoga postures for promoting good health and strengthening the internal organs.

There are many benefits to inversions. It has been scientifically proven that when men either stand on their heads or lean on their heads over the edge of a bed for at least fifteen seconds per day, hair growth is stimulated. The ancient Yoga masters knew this thousands of years ago. By defying gravity you can reverse the effects of aging and improve your overall health.

Lymph, a clear yellowish fluid that circulates through the body, is pulled down by gravity during the course of a day. Inversions clear the lymphatic passageways and revitalize the entire body. The positive effects of inversions on the endocrine system include

1. Ability to face fears
2. More positive approach to life

3. Lucidity and creativity

4. Longevity

Before doing an inversion there are some things to consider. To protect your neck, you should precede these postures with the Opening Bell (Sun Salutation) outlined in Chapter 5. Do not attempt an inversion if you have high blood pressure, hiatus hernia, glaucoma, or neck problems. In addition, if you are overweight use your best judgment. Also use caution if you are balancing against a mirrored or glass surface. Inversions will be explained in detail in Chapter 4. To reduce the possibility of light-headedness, start out slowly and gradually increase the time you hold your positions.

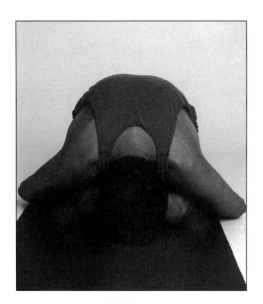

FIGURE 4.5

After an inversion it is recommended that you assume the Child's Pose. (See Figure 4.5.)

1. Kneel on your hands and knees, with your knees hip width apart, and your hands below your shoulders.

2. As you exhale, sit back onto your heels, keeping the tops of your feet flat on the floor. Bend forward at the hips with your chest on your thighs and your forehead on the floor.

3. Lay your arms on the floor beside your torso, palms up.

4. Close your eyes and breathe slowly and gently.

You should try to remain in all positions for at least 30 seconds. You can gradually increase the length of time you hold a pose. If you feel any pain or discomfort, discontinue immediately.

Twists

Twists are very important for strengthening the spine, improving circulation, and massaging internal organs. Unfortunately, for people with disk problems, these exercises are not appropriate. (See Figure 4.6.)

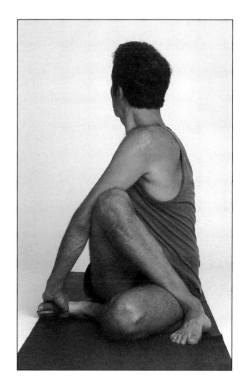

FIGURE 4.6

CHAPTER FIVE

Basic Yoga Workout

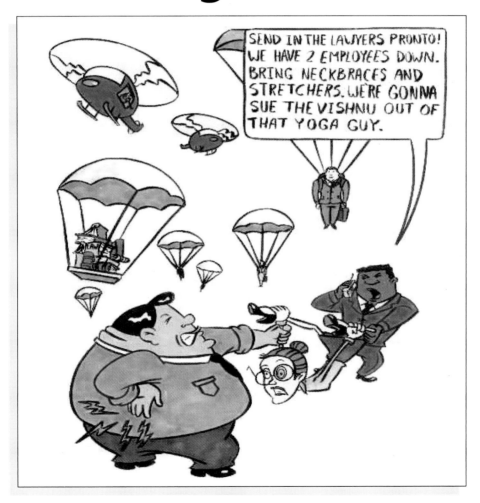

Manny Problemas, Marketing Manager, Ann Thracks, Accounting
Manager, Oscar Fodder, Operations Manager, End Run Corporation

This chapter outlines a recommended daily Yoga workout routine that provides a complete physical workout. I have renamed positions in Yoga using terms from business to help you identify with the movement and focus your attention. The corresponding Yogic terminology is also given, along with the physiological benefits.

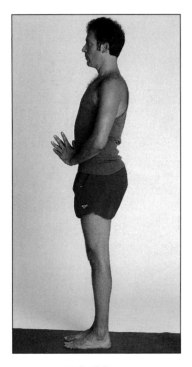

FIGURE 5.1

1. Opening Bell (Sun Salutation)

Time: 5 to 10 minutes
(at least 30 seconds in each position if possible)

Benefits: Energizing after rest, improved circulation

Keep your knees a little soft. Be sure your buttocks are contracted slightly, your spinal column long, and your head, neck, and shoulders completely relaxed.

a. Standing with your eyes closed, feet about five inches apart, and hands together in a prayerful attitude, begin to feel the breath flowing gently into your lungs and imagine it filling your belly, ribs, and chest with fresh air. (See Figure 5.1.) Take a moment to dedicate this practice as a time for yourself as you bring your hands together. Lift your hands toward the heavens. Think to yourself as you inhale, I hold my ground while I remain flexible to change. Today I will stretch my body, mind, and creativity. (See Figure 5.2.)

b. As you reach the apex, allow your arms to separate and arch backward, stretching your spinal column and lifting your sternum.

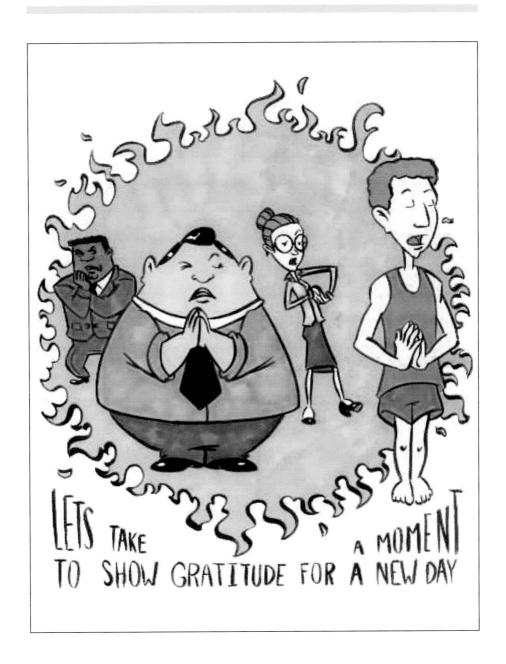

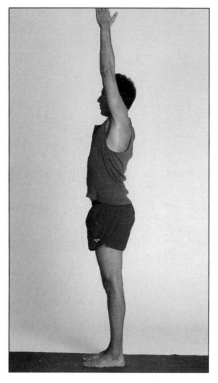

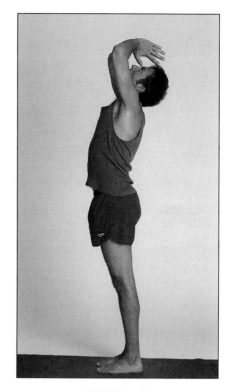

| FIGURE 5.2 | FIGURE 5.3 |

Make sure to soften your shoulders away from your ears as you exhale. (See Figure 5.3.)

c. Reach up and lean back slightly to stretch as you inhale. Then, on the exhalation, begin to hinge forward slowly from the hips to allow your torso to fall forward and your hands to fall toward your feet. Simply surrender to gravity and release. Keep breathing deeply. Notice any areas of resistance, and direct the breath into these areas.

Modification: If your legs are tight or you have lower back pain, bend your knees as you hinge forward.

d. As you continue to exhale, place your hands by the sides of your feet and soften your knees if needed. (See Figure 5.4.)

e. Inhale, step back with your right leg, and rest your right knee and shin on the floor. Allow your hands and right knee to keep your balance. Your left foot supports your weight. Release the pelvis forward and down to help gravity extend the stretch and open your groin. Relax your jaw and face. Keep your left foot and both hands connected firmly to the earth. Breathe smoothly. (See Figure 5.5.)

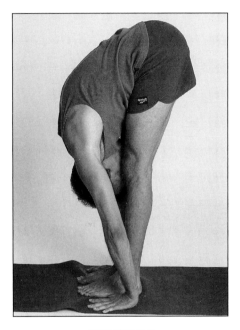

f. Exhale and step back with your left leg to a push-up position while supporting the weight of your torso with your hands. Press out through your heels and engage your abdominal muscles so your back doesn't sway. (See Figure 5.6.)

Modification: If your arms give out, then bring your knees to the floor for support.

FIGURE 5.4

g. Inhale, then exhale. Press your hips up to form a triangle. Push your buttocks back and lengthen your spine by dropping your chest toward your knees, keeping your hands firmly rooted down. Try to press your head toward the floor and lift your buttocks toward the ceiling. (See Figure 5.7.)

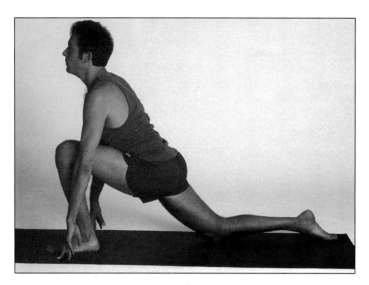

FIGURE 5.5

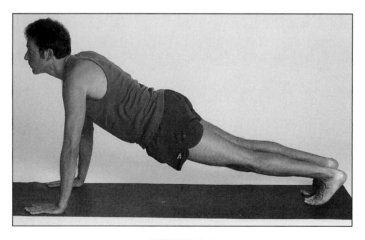

FIGURE 5.6

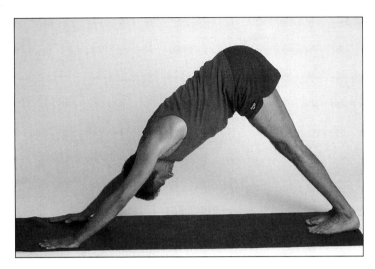

FIGURE 5.7

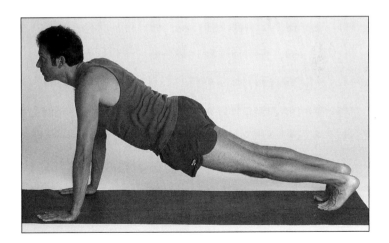

FIGURE 5.8

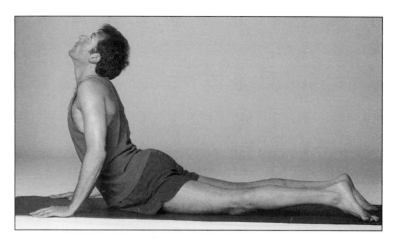

FIGURE 5.9

If you are having trouble getting your heels to the floor, don't worry. It takes time to get the hamstrings to loosen and elongate.

h. Inhale. Then exhale back into a plank or push-up position. (See Figure 5.8.)

i. Inhale, and begin to feel the pressure on your hands as you slide your chest along the floor, raising your upper torso, arching your back, and pressing your chest forward while keeping your pelvis connected to the floor. Lower your shoulders away from your neck. Your legs are outstretched and the tops of your feet are on the floor. Keep your belly button and lower abdomen connected to the floor. Keep your chest open. Push away from the floor as you draw your elbows and shoulder blades back. Like a cobra, open your heart center and throat. Exhale and continue normal breathing during the duration of this exercise. (See Figure 5.9.)

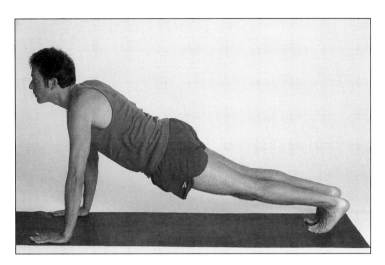

FIGURE 5.10

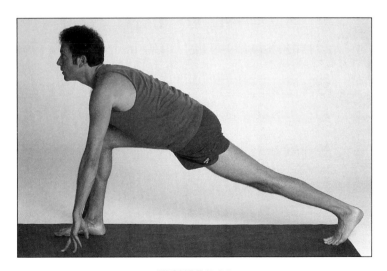

FIGURE 5.11

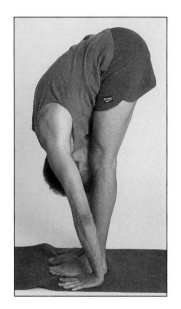

FIGURE 5.12

j. Inhale, then turn your feet so you are back on your toes. Exhale back into a push-up position. (See Figure 5.10.)

k. On the inhalation, step forward with your right leg, this time keeping your left knee off the floor. With your right foot planted firmly on the floor, keep your left leg extended and your weight on your toes. Allow your hands and feet to support your body. Try to extend the stretch by allowing gravity to carry your pelvis even lower. Exhale and continue to breathe deeply to open your groin. Relax your jaw and face, and breathe smoothly. (See Figure 5.11.)

l. On the inhalation, step forward with your left leg bent until you are in a bent-over stretch. Keep your knees slightly soft. Turn the under part of your sitting bones up to the ceiling. Let your spine elongate, your neck be soft, and your face relax. Surrender to earth and gravity. (See Figure 5.12.) Engage your abdominal muscles, straighten your back, and slowly let your body rise to greet a new day. Begin to reach up toward the heavens and bring your hands to your sides. (See Figure 5.13.)

Repeat the entire sequence, reversing the left and right positions, as you exhale and then continue normal breathing.

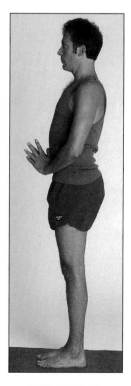

FIGURE 5.13

2. Maximizing Resources (Kapalabhati) Pranayama

Time: 30 to 60 seconds

Benefits: Increased mental alertness, emotional balance, improved digestion, abdominal muscle development, energy

Sit with your legs crossed in the Easy Posture. (If you are stiff—your hips are not rotating and your knees are high—see the suggestions on page 38.

You may want to begin by putting your hand on your belly to learn the art of breathing deeply from the abdomen. Start off by gently breathing in slow motion, lengthening the inhalation and exhalation each time. Then increase the speed, focusing on forcing the air out of your nostrils in short breaths. The inhalation will occur naturally.

As you get more comfortable with this exercise, begin to tighten your sphincter muscles on the exhalation.

Keep your face, shoulders, and chest relaxed. Continue forcing air out of your lungs in quick motions for at least 60 seconds.

If you find yourself getting dizzy, exhale into your hand and relax for a few minutes. This pose is called Maximizing Resources because you are filling your body with more oxygen, a resource you may not have been using to its full and necessary extent. This exercise will clear your sinuses and bring more oxygen to your brain, stimulating brain cells. It will also strengthen your abdominal muscles and massage your internal organs.

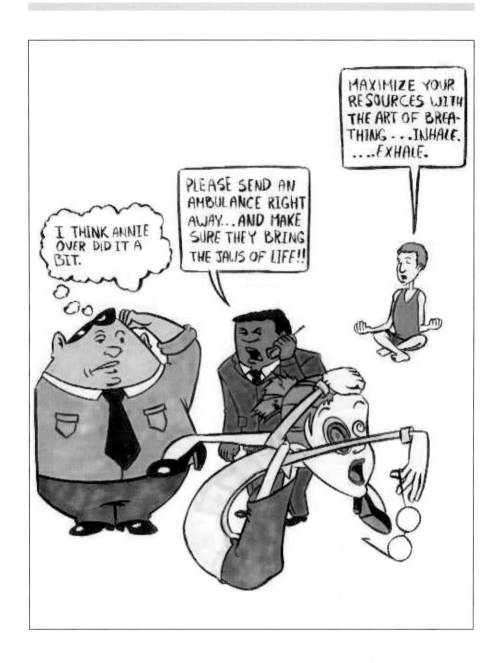

3. Strategic Alignment (Alternate Leg Stretch)

Time: 30 to 60 seconds

Benefits: Strength and increased flexibility in spine, improved circulation, alleviation of constipation, energizing of lymphatic system

Extend your legs in front of you, leaving about twelve inches between them. Sit firmly and evenly on your sitting bones. Bend your left knee, and bring the bottom of your left foot in to touch the inside of your right thigh. For those tight in the hips, the bent knee will be quite a distance from the ground, so use pillows to balance your sitting bones. Prepare for this position by lifting through your spine, visualizing the spine as an accordion. First open the accordion by stretching upward, slightly twist to the left and attempt to touch your knee with your forehead, then bend forward. Use your arms to stretch upward first and then twist slightly forward over the extended right leg. Be sure that the center of your chest is directly over the center of your outstretched

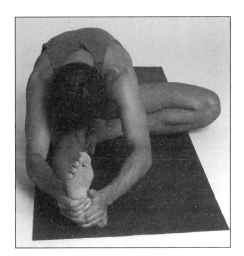

FIGURE 5.14

leg. Feel a twist through your left hip. Exhale as you stretch over your bent left leg, drive your left buttock back into the floor and breathe into the position. With each exhalation, surrender into a deeper stretch, allowing the breath to bring you to your absolute maximum in the posture. (See Figure 5.14.)

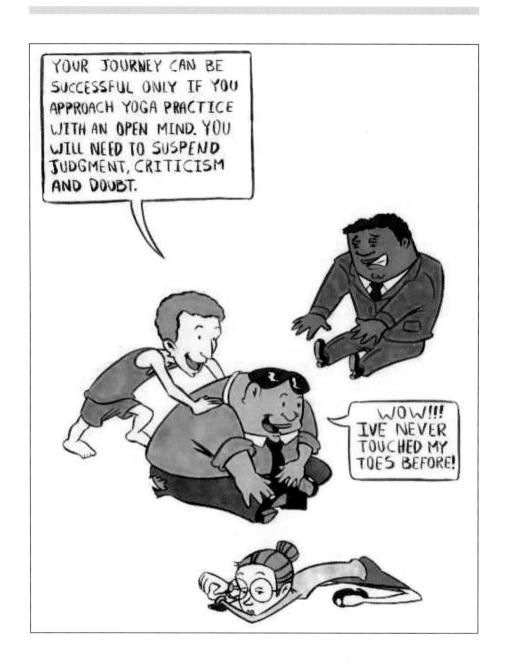

On the opposite side of the stretch, your right knee is bent and your right foot placed along the inside of your left thigh.

There are three keys to this pose:

1. Stretch up.

2. Twist slightly.

3. Extend and center.

4. Downsizing the Middle (Sit-ups and Scissors)

Time: 30 to 60 seconds for each

Benefits: Improved breathing, abdominal muscle development

Breathing exercises support movement, and abdominal exercise can be used as a backdrop for learning how to breathe. Two benefits will occur. First, you will become less focused on the quantity of repetitions and more focused on the breath. This shift of focus allows you to do more. If your abdominal muscles are weak, make sure that your lower back is flush with the floor. Be certain that your hands are interlaced behind your head, and that they support the head, not the neck, to protect the upper back. For those not in very good shape, start by extending one leg on the floor and doing individual leg lifts. Once you feel more confident, you can move on to the next step.

PEDALING

Lie flat on your back on the floor. With your hands behind your head for support, raise your right elbow and your left knee. Attempt to bring them together on the exhalation. Lower slowly on the inhalation and

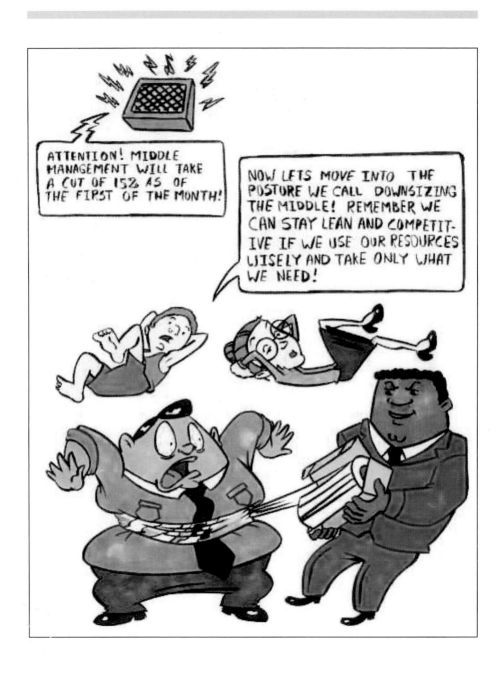

repeat on the opposite side. Continue with the breath and build up to 60 seconds. (See Figure 5.15.)

SCISSORS

Lay flat on your back on the floor. With your hands at your sides, attempt to raise your feet about six inches off the ground. Cross your legs right over left on the exhalation and left over right on the inhalation. Continue with the breath and build up to 60 seconds.

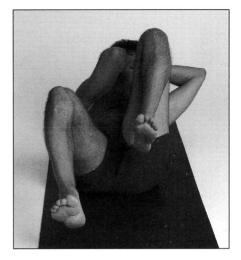

FIGURE 5.15

5. Firm Footing in a Changing Marketplace (Warrior Pose/Tree Pose)

Time: 30 to 60 seconds on each leg

Benefits: Balanced left- and right-brain functioning, mental stability, relief of addictions and depression, strengthening of legs, hips, and feet

WARRIOR POSE

Like an Olympic diver about to make a dive, keep your eyes unfocused and go within. Stand on your right leg and spread your toes as wide as possible to make as much contact with the floor as you can. Visualize this foot as a snowshoe. Extend your left leg back slowly and point the toe. Exhale as your torso begins to fold forward, raise

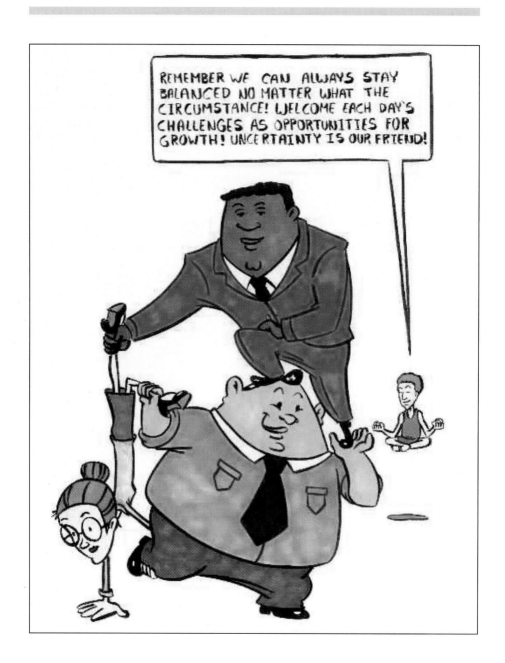

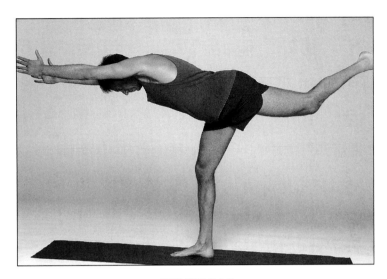

FIGURE 5.16

your arms alongside your ears, keeping your fingers together and extended, projecting the energy field outward. You will feel like a strip of energy extending from the tips of your fingers through your body to your feet, pulling and strengthening your lumbar spine (lower back). Align your hips. Your gaze should be forward and shortly down. Your breathing should be slow and regular. A steady gaze will help you maintain steadiness. Your right leg should act like a tall, strong tree with your arms like branches. Remember that nothing can shake you from the foundation of your inner strength and source of power. If you can, hold this position for 30 seconds. (See Figure 5.16.) When you come out, slowly lower your left leg, holding your hands together at the heart. Bring yourself to a vertical position, standing tall with hands together at prayer position, for 30 seconds of deep relaxing breath. Repeat on the other side.

TREE POSE

Stand in an upright position. Inhale, raise your arms, and stretch upward. Lift your right foot off the floor. If you are comfortable with your balance, bend your right knee, raise it toward your chest, and support your left leg by placing the right foot against the inside of the left thigh. (See Figure 5.17.) Hold this position, then repeat on the other side. If you feel less secure, do this exercise near a wall or a piece of furniture that you can use for support. In the beginning you may want to practice balancing on one foot, with your other foot just slightly off the floor. Build to 60 seconds on each leg.

The following position is advanced and should not be attempted if you have any medical conditions.

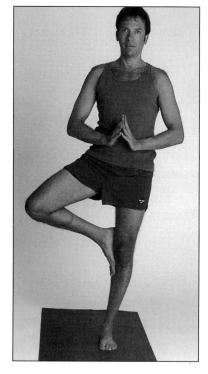

FIGURE 5.17

6. Change from the Top Down (Headstand Pose)

Time: 30 to 60 seconds

Benefits: Tonification of the vital organs; stimulation of endocrine glands; reduced male pattern baldness; reversal of the aging process; total upper body conditioning; abdominal conditioning; greater strength and elasticity in superficial and deep musculature, ligaments, and connective tissue of the spine and rib cage; improved posture and overall structural integrity of the body, better digestion, respiration, and circulation

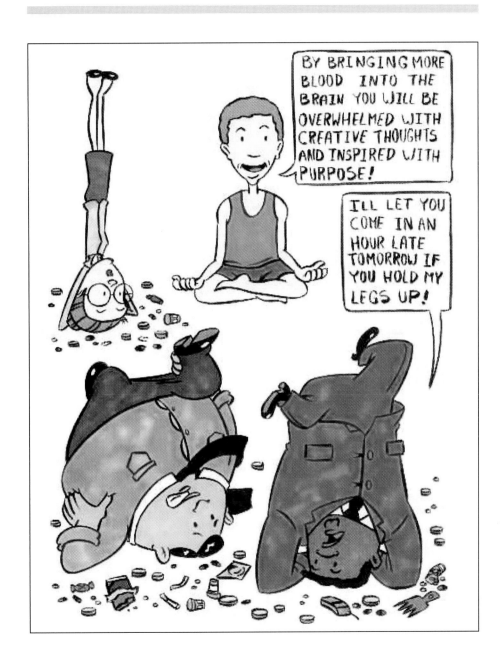

Assume the Child's Pose on the floor, preferably in front of a wall, which can support you if you fall backward. (See Figure 4.5.) Make sure there is ample padding from a mat, some pillows, or a folded-up blanket. Clasp your hands behind your head and make sure your fingers are interlaced around the back of the head. Your elbows should be shoulder width apart. Gently place your head on the floor. Inhale as you gently walk your feet toward your head. Slowly lift up into the

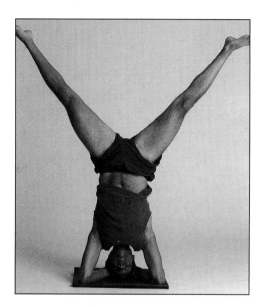

FIGURE 5.18

headstand, attempting to keep lifting, bringing the energy up so you're not collapsed into the position. (See Figure 5.18.) Breathing normally and supporting your weight with your forearms and the strength of your shoulders, feel the blood circulating through your brain cells, stimulating, restoring, reversing aging, oxygenating the upper portions of your body, releasing pressure on the lower organs and the legs, clearing the veins, and redirecting the flow of lymph. Hold the pose for 30 to 60 seconds, or as long as possible, then gently lower your feet back to the floor.

Modification: Follow the procedure just outlined, but raise the right, then the left leg. In a kneeling position, clasp hands around the head and straighten legs to get your torso perpendicular to the ground. Beginners should not focus on raising the legs but on getting comfortable in the pose and strengthening the arms.

7. Bending Over Backward to Serve Your Customers (Camel Pose)

Time: 30 to 60 seconds

Benefits: Stretching of abdominal organs, relieving visceral compression; gentle massage of kidney and adrenal area, stimulating and improving its functioning; stretching of neck and throat, massaging thyroid and thymus glands; strengthening of torso, shoulder, pelvic girdle, and leg musculature

On your knees (with toes curled under and heels elevated for beginners), slowly bend your torso and head backward while pushing your

chest forward. Your hands are supporting your weight by holding your feet at the heels. Your thighs rotate in while your hips press forward. Your sternum should be lifted high to avoid compression in your neck. As you reach farther back for the heels or soles of your feet, draw your shoulder blades together tightly and keep your shoulders down. On the inhalation, extend your chest up and forward, feeling the rib cage opening and making space for the energy of the heart chakra. Extend your pelvis forward so your focus is not bending back but pushing forward. Bending back is incidental to this position. (See Figure 5.19.) When you are ready, come out of the position by gently releasing your hands and leading your head,

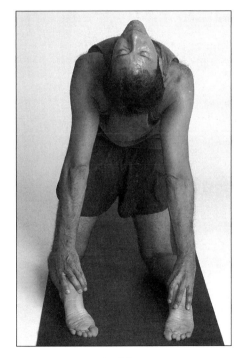

FIGURE 5.19

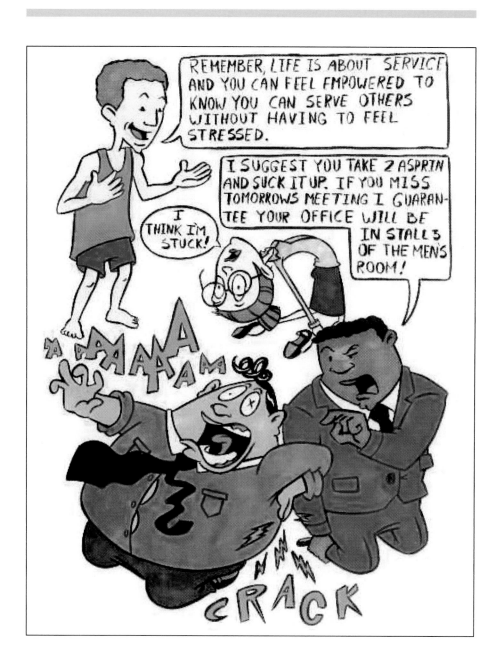

then your upper body, forward and down into Child's Pose for a brief rest. (See Figure 4.5.)

Modification: An easier variation of this exercise is to position yourself with a chair or bed behind you, so you can create an arch without having to extend your back fully. Extend your arms behind you to support your arch using the furniture.

8. Deflating a Bloated Bureaucracy (Ashivini Mudra/Mula Bandha)

Time: 30 to 60 seconds

Benefits: Emotional balancing, clarity of mental processes, improved digestion and burning of food and calories, better circulation to the kidneys, enhanced sexual performance, stamina, and heightened orgasm, strengthens prostrate region, preventing prostate conditions.

Get down on your hands and knees to practice this breathing/pelvic stimulation exercise. It is helpful to imagine a square block between your arms and thighs so that the arms and thighs are perpendicular to the floor and ceiling. On the inhalation, press your chest forward and arch your pelvis back. (See Figure 5.20.) On the exhalation, make your chest concave and tilt your pelvis forward. (See Figure 5.21.) At that point engage and lift the anus and prostate muscles. The alternating motion looks like arching waves. Remember to be gentle with your neck. Continue for 60 seconds if you can, with 4 seconds of inhalation to 8 seconds of exhalation, if possible.

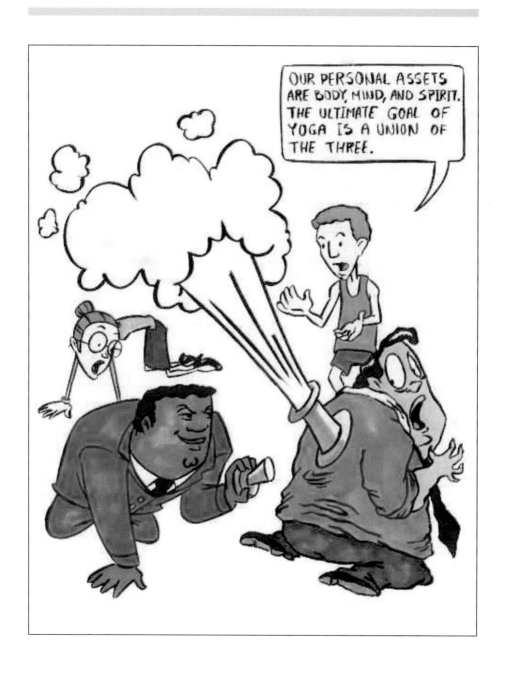

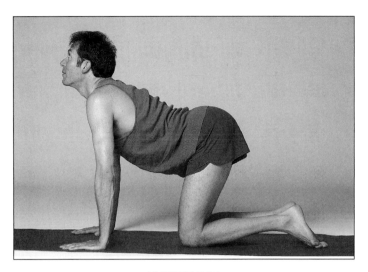

FIGURE 5.20

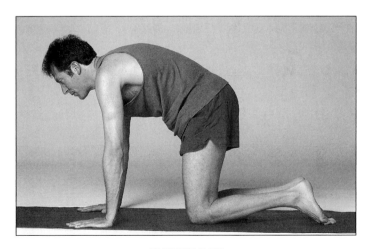

FIGURE 5.21

Caution: This position is advanced and should not be attempted if you have any medical conditions.

9. Bridging Corporate Cultures (Wheel Pose)

Time: 30 to 60 seconds

Benefits: Stretching of abdominal organs, relieving visceral compression; gentle massaging of kidney and adrenal area, stimulating and improving its functioning; stretching of neck and throat, massaging thyroid and thymus glands; strengthening of torso, shoulder, and pelvic girdle, and leg musculature

Lay flat on your back and raise your hips. Inhale as you push your torso up by lifting your weight onto your arms and extending forward in the direction of your gaze. Feel the strengthening in your

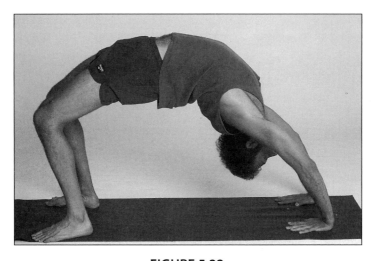

FIGURE 5.22

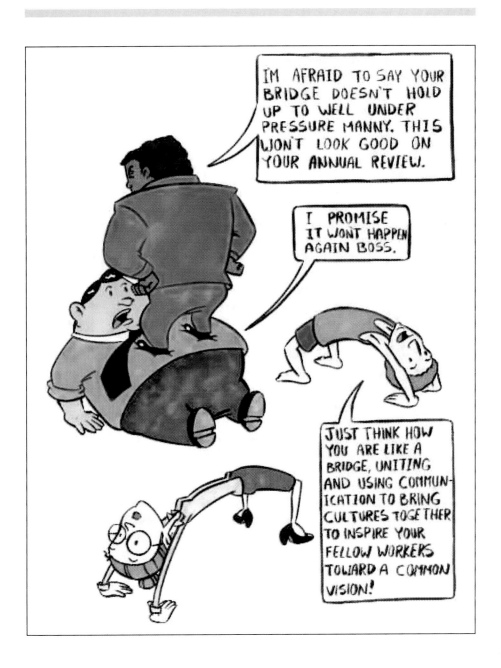

arms. Lift as high and as far forward as your chest will allow and breathe normally. (See Figure 5.22.) As you slowly lower your body, attempt to lift your head and tuck your chin so that the lower back portion of your head is cradled against the floor. In a full back bend the interior of the spinal column stimulates all the nerve passages. After you come back to a resting pose, flat on your back, draw your knees into your chest as a counterpose so your spinal cord stretches in the opposite direction.

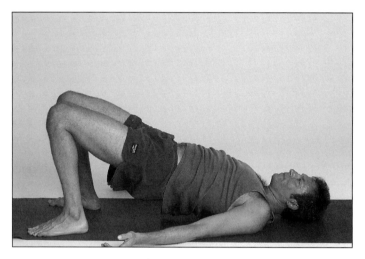

FIGURE 5.23

Caution: Do not move your neck while in this position.

Modification: Lying flat on your back, extend your arms beside your body. Using your arms for leverage, raise your torso with your legs only. Use the muscles in the thighs and buttocks to support your weight. (See Figure 5.23.)

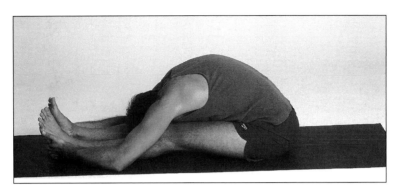

FIGURE 5.24

10. Redeploying Assets (Forward Stretch)

Time: 30 to 60 seconds

Benefits: Strength and increased flexibility in spine, improved circulation, alleviation of constipation, energizing of lymphatic system

Sit upright on your sitting bones with your legs stretched out in front of you. Extend your arms, reaching for your toes, and exhale into the extension, opening the sinews of your sciatic nerves. Exhale deeply, attempting to lower yourself farther, and direct your energy between your eyebrows. Direct your energy into the areas that resist the most. Feel your tension dissolving as you surrender to gravity. (See Figure 5.24.) When you are ready, release and come up slowly. Shake out your legs to jump-start circulation.

Modification: Beginners should use support, such as a pillow or folded blanket, under the buttocks. Also use caution if you have lower back pain or a herniated disk.

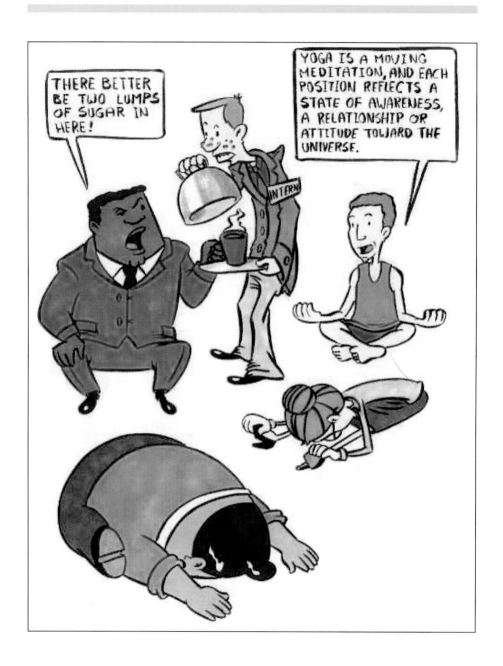

11. Timing Acquisitions (Breathing Arches)

Time: 30 to 60 seconds

Benefits: Increased mental alertness, emotional balance, improved digestion, abdominal muscle development

Begin in a seated position comfortable for you, preferably with your legs crossed. With your hands using your shins as levers, start flexing your spine back and forth, taking inhalations on the forward motion (see Figure 5.25) and exhalations on the reverse (see Figure 5.26). Stay focused on keeping your shoulders down. With each inhalation extend your chest higher and fuller, drawing your shoulder blades down and closer together. Continue for 60 seconds if possible. Then relax in your seated position.

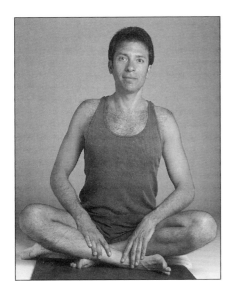

FIGURE 5.25

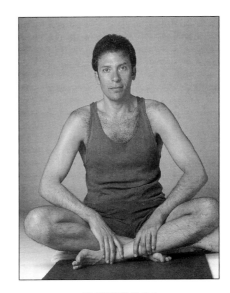

FIGURE 5.26

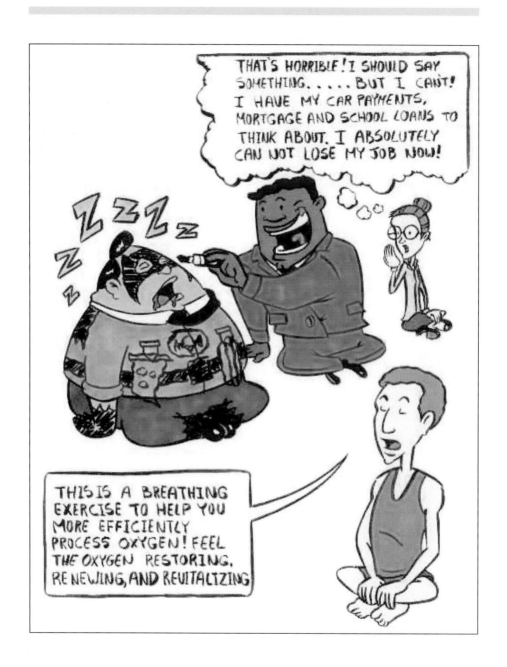

12. Global Vision (Spinal Twist)

Time: 30 to 60 seconds on each side

Benefits: Improved strength and elasticity of spinal column, stimulating respiratory organs and functioning, and massaging liver, kidneys, adrenals, gallbladder, pancreas, and spleen; compressing and stretching of intestines, stimulating the absorption, digestion, and elimination functions; improved balance; increased strength in upper body, shoulders, and pelvic girdle

Begin by sitting in the Easy Posture. (See Figure 4.2.) Take your right leg and place it over your left. Twist your torso to the right. Your right hand should be behind your back to provide additional support. Your left hand serves as a lever, helping you twist to full capacity. Exhale as you continue to stretch and push at your hips, twisting, not grinding. (See Figure 5.27.)

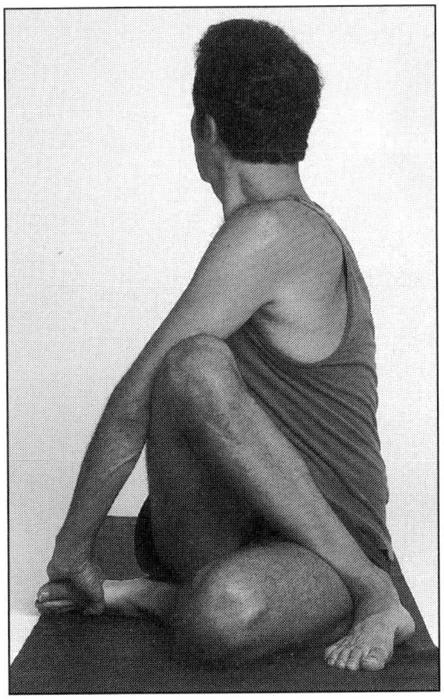

Attempt to keep your sitting bones evenly on the floor. Try to resist the temptation to lift one side of your buttocks to give a better stretch. This will throw your spine out of alignment. Also try not to lean on your hand too much. Remember that the spine is an accordion, which must be extended first. Create space between each pair of vertebrae and disks, with emphasis on vertically extending the spine, then twist slowly. During exhalation, attempt to twist a little farther. Slowly come out of the position by reversing the twist and returning to your initial seated position. Repeat on the other side.

FIGURE 5.27

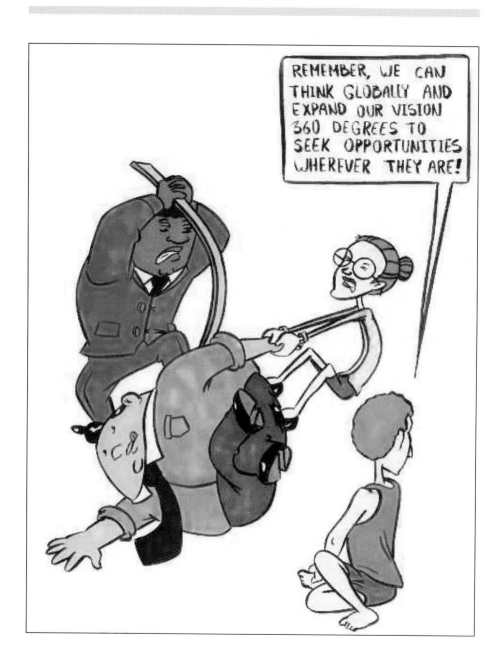

Caution: This is an advanced position and should be attempted only by individuals who are very athletic and have a lot of upper body strength. If you have any neck problems, consult your physician before attempting this exercise. In addition, do not attempt to move your neck while in this position.

13. Shouldering Responsibility (Handstand/Shoulder Stand)

Time: 15 to 30 seconds

Benefits: Tonification of the vital organs, stimulation of the endocrine gland, reduced male pattern baldness, reversal of the aging process, total upper body conditioning, abdominal conditioning, greater strength and elasticity in the superficial and deep musculature, ligaments, and connective tissue of the spine and rib cage; improved posture, and overall structural integrity, promoting better digestion, respiration, and circulation, stimulation of endocrine glands

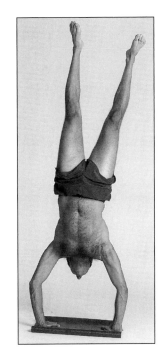

Bend over next to a wall and put your weight on your hands and arms. Inhale as you gently kick each leg upward into a handstand pose, allowing the wall to stop you at a vertical position. Your hands are spread and your feet are straight. Flex your feet a little, pushing the toes up. This lifts the lower back–sacrum area. (See Figure 5.28.) When you are ready, slowly lower your legs onto the floor and sit in the Easy Posture. (See Figure 4.2.)

FIGURE 5.28

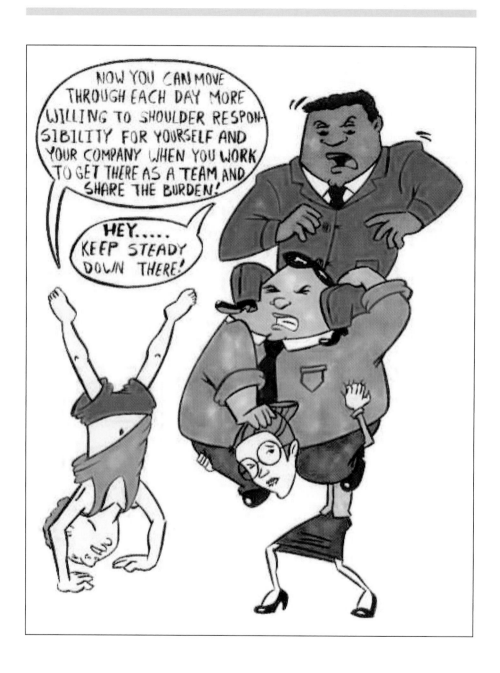

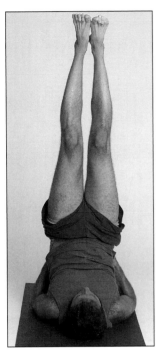

FIGURE 5.29

Modification: Position yourself on a mat with your buttocks against a wall. Place two or three folded blankets beneath your buttocks. Raise your hips and support your weight with your hands. Position your legs against the wall for balance. (See Figure 5.29.) After a month or so you may be able to straighten your legs without using the wall. After several months you can lengthen the position by lifting more fully into a full shoulder stand.

Meditation

Time: 15 to 30 minutes

Benefits: Slows aging process, promotes healing in the body, improves focus, mental clarity, and problem-solving ability

Give yourself the gift of space and time to cool down. Meditation is the natural practice of withdrawing attention from the external world, including physical and mental processes, and consciously directing it inward to a chosen focus or concentration. Imagine a favorite spot that is special to you. Bring those feelings to your body and rejoice in a new day. Yoga has now allowed you to quiet your body; meditation will quiet your mind. So if you're able, sit on the floor with your legs crossed and back straight. If you're in a chair, sit upright and close your eyes. (See Figure 5.30.) If your mind wanders, gently bring

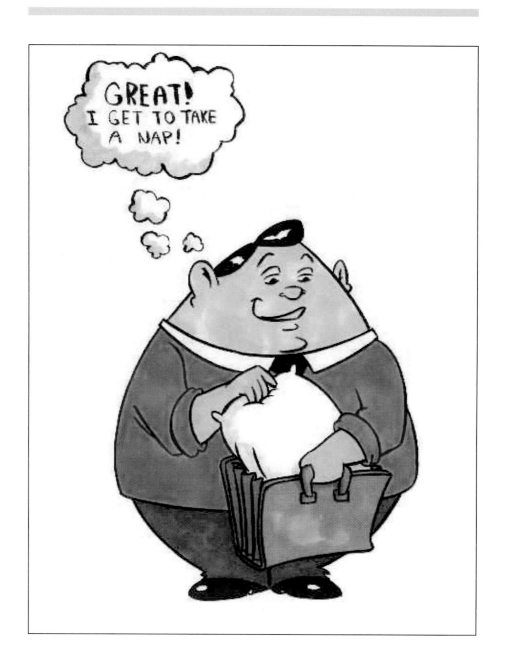

it back to your breathing. In meditation you will learn you are not your thoughts; you are the thinker who has the thoughts. But for now quiet those thoughts.

Place your hands on your lower abdomen and listen to the breath as it rises and falls. As you continue breathing deeply, you'll find yourself relaxing more and more with each breath.

Here is a series of suggested images for your meditation. You may want to first read the following text and then listen to it on the CD to help you focus. Or simply call to mind this or similar serene imagery that will help you block out all distracting thoughts.

STREAM MEDITATION

The stream starts out deep within the earth, as an underground spring in a glacial mountain, and bubbles up through levels of sediment and rock, finally emerging as pure, sparkling water that has its own form but also reflects the images of the world. It is illuminated by the warmth of the sun.

As the stream, you can re-create yourself daily and flow more easily through the rapids. In fact you may enjoy the rapids, noticing how the air is electrified and purified by the water molecules colliding and dancing, their subatomic particles twirling at lightning speed.

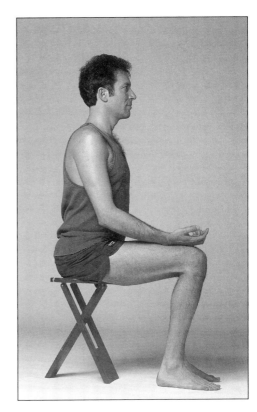

FIGURE 5.30

You can now move through the rapids and feel exhilarated and enlivened without having to feel squeezed, burdened, or stressed. Each day you can flow through life with more confidence, knowing that you are the master of the stream, because you no longer will be caught. There will always be parts of the stream where the land is less forgiving, but now you flow through them more balanced and centered, knowing that they are just transitions that always lead to growth. Every stream widens after the rapids, and there is an abundance of life renewing and restoring after the turbulent waters.

Some streams end their journeys in a lake or pond, but you join others to form a river, sharing the experience, knowledge, and information you have acquired from your journey; in turn you receive valuable insights and assistance from others, and in this exchange of giving and receiving there is balance. And by combining strengths, and sharing experience and effort, all participants can reach the sea.

As you flow out into the sea with all the streams that have joined you to form a river and all the rivers that are now flowing with you into unity, you feel open and spacious. As the ocean you are free, unbounded and infinite. Linger here a moment. Notice that your normal sense of time and space is irrelevant here. The gentle ebb and flow of the water and the movement of light creates a feeling of suspended time, or timelessness. Maybe you are watching magnificent whales frolicking; maybe you are swimming beside them. Or you might be captivated by the brilliant colors of the coral reefs, with their interesting shapes and designs and thousands of fish, noticing how by some divine intelligence a school of fish moves in unison, and how life proceeds naturally and effortlessly without your intervention. Or you may be mesmerized by the ebb and flow of the tides and how the seaweed and plant growth moves so gracefully. And you are aware that your breath is flowing in unison with the motion of the tide because you are the sea. So the natural rhythms of life can bring you back here at any time, for all you have to do is breathe deeply and repeat, I am the stream. I am the river. I am the ocean.

When you are ready, slowly become aware of your body and come back into this place, feeling refreshed and ready for the challenges of the day.

CHAPTER SIX

Yoga Practices to Improve Prostate Health and Sexual Performance

Here are some winning strategies you can use to protect your health and improve sexual performance.

1. Energize and recharge your body daily with Yoga practice. In this chapter, Yoga positions that are extremely useful in opening and strengthening the second chakra region will be discussed.

2. Breathe deeply and more frequently during the day.

3. Change your belief systems. Individuals who are able to paint a compelling picture of health in their minds can live a life with passion.

4. Heal your sexual relationships. Sexual union can be achieved even without orgasm. Many men think that the objective of sex is an orgasm, but a survivor will tell you that a healing and spiritual union is the real goal. Exercises such as meditation on unconditional love will be discussed as a way to make the sexual experience less tense and decrease the pressure to perform.

5. Extend your sexual arousal through Tantra Yoga. With the pressure of performance gone and the breathing exercises you will learn, you can extend and heighten the sexual healing experience. This chapter will discuss how to move energy up from the base of the spine to the crown of your head.

6. Share energy healing with your partner. Reiki, which is universal life energy, can energize you and put you in the moment, which to most people means "in the mood." We will discuss some Reiki positions you can use with your significant other.

7. Love yourself more.

8. Eat right.

Postures to Improve Sexual Performance

The energy boost you can receive from Yoga will improve your sexual performance naturally and more effectively.

The Deflating a Bloated Bureaucracy exercise (see page 69) will help to open energy pathways in the body that have been blocked. In men this exercise contributes to the health of the prostate and offers more control over ejaculation. Gaining control of your breathing and being in the moment will not only improve your sexual stamina but also create a much more sensual and meaningful experience of union.

If you have serious medical problems with your urogenital tract, consult a physician before doing these exercises.

KEGEL EXERCISES

The Kegel exercises, which were derived from Yoga, are breathing–muscle contraction exercises that strengthen the pelvic floor. They squeeze the sphincter muscle. You can practice these exercises while you are urinating to get familiar with the sensation. I recommend doing these exercises throughout the day.

Caution: If you are experiencing any pain in the prostate area, please consult with your physician before attempting these exercises.

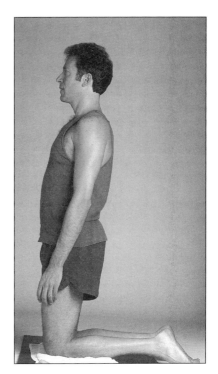

FIGURE 6.1

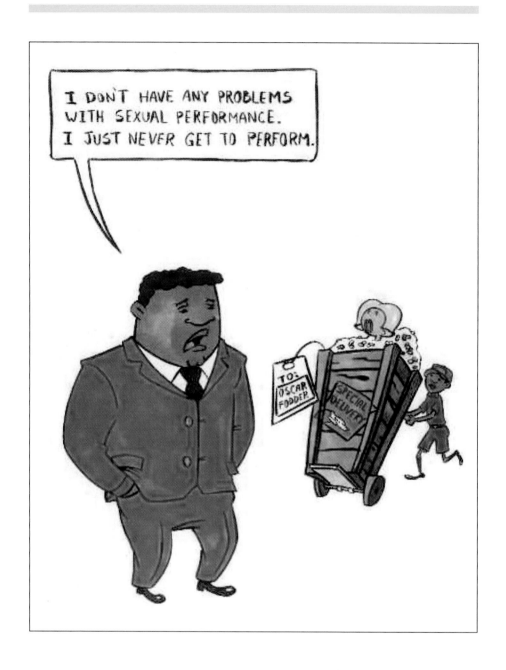

Sit up in your chair, wherever you may be. Take a few deep breaths, and on the exhalation begin to contract your sphincter muscle. Try ten quick inhalations and exhalations, then make the last cycle a long, deep inhalation and hold the exhalation contraction for 10 seconds.

The most effective way to perform the Kegel exercises is in the Frog Pose. For this position you will need three blankets.

Frog Pose

Time: 30 to 60 seconds

Benefits: Opening and strengthening of pelvic region and prostate gland, improved sexual functioning

Fold the first blanket and kneel on top of it. (See Figure 6.1.)

Roll the other two blankets and place them on top of your calves. Now lower your buttocks onto the blankets to a comfortable seated position. (See Figure 6.2.)

Rise slowly when you are finished with the Kegel exercises and stretch your legs.

Body Drops are another floor exercise that targets the acupressure points related to the prostate.

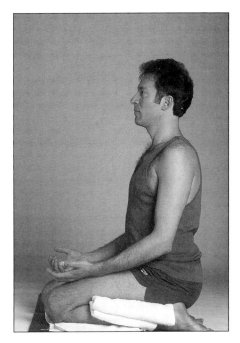

FIGURE 6.2

Body Drops

Time: 30 to 60 seconds

Benefits: Opening and strengthening of pelvic region
and prostate gland, improved sexual functioning

Position yourself on your mat with your legs outstretched and your torso, neck, and head aligned. (See Figure 6.3.)

Put your arms at your sides, palms on the floor, and begin to lift your torso. Your hands and feet support your weight. (See Figure 6.4.)

Now lower yourself gently to the floor and repeat.

The Locust Pose, or Bow Pose, is also an effective overall method of strengthening the lower back and nervous system, and increasing circulation to the pelvic region.

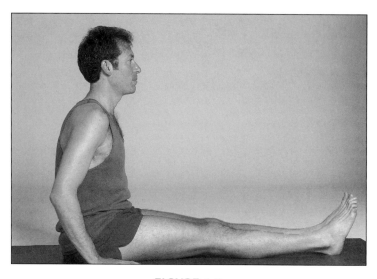

FIGURE 6.3

Caution: If you have lower back pain, please consult with your physician before doing this exercise.

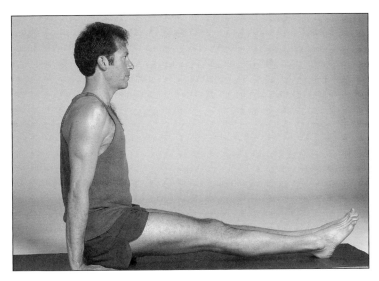

FIGURE 6.4

Locust Pose (Bow Pose)

Time: 30 to 60 seconds

Benefits: Opening and strengthening of pelvic region and prostate gland, improved sexual functioning

Lie chest down on your mat with your arms along your sides, palms up. (See Figure 6.5.) The weight of your head is resting on your chin and your toes are extended. Your breathing is relaxed.

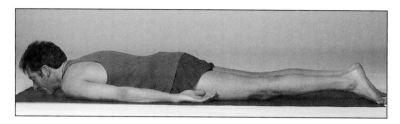

FIGURE 6.5

Inhale as you engage your thighs and calves. Tighten your buttocks as you simultaneously raise your legs, arms, head, neck, and finally chest. If you are able, hold for up to 30 seconds. As you breathe slowly your palms should be facing upward and your gaze should be forward and unfocused. (See Figure 6.6.) When finished, slowly lower your upper and lower body in unison and exhale. Repeat as many times as possible.

Caution: If you have any lower back pain, please consult with your physician before doing this exercise.

The Fish Pose with Frog's Legs is a combination that will not only provide relaxation but also improve the flow of oxygen and circulation in the body, and open the first and second chakras.

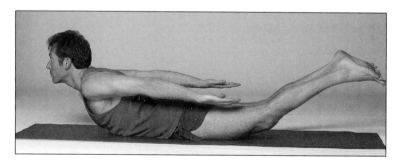

FIGURE 6.6

Fish Pose with Frog's Legs

Time: 30 to 60 seconds

Benefits: Strengthening of neck, improved respiration, opening and strengthening of pelvic region and prostate gland, improved sexual functioning

Sit on your mat with your legs outstretched in front of you and your head, neck, and torso aligned. Your hands are resting on your lap, palms are facing upward, and breathing is normal and relaxed. Place about four folded blankets right behind your buttocks. (See Figure 6.7.)

Slowly lower your back toward the mat and place your hands under your buttocks. (See Figure 6.8.)

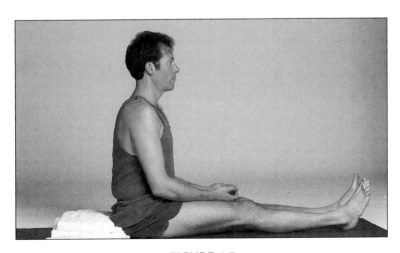

FIGURE 6.7

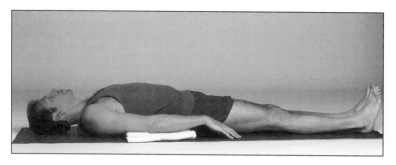

FIGURE 6.8

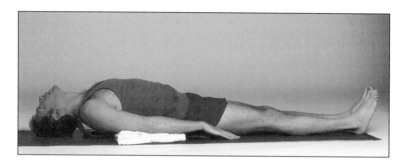

FIGURE 6.9

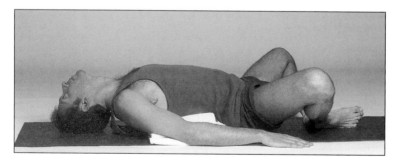

FIGURE 6.10

Bend your neck slightly backward to accentuate the arch formed by your body across the cushion of blankets. (See Figure 6.9.)

Now bend your knees and put your heels together. Allow gravity and your breath to spread your legs and open your groin as much as possible. Hold for 30 seconds if possible. (See Figure 6.10.) Release by stretching your legs out in front of you and slowly coming up to a seated posture.

I also recommend the Plank (Push-up) Position and the Cobra Pose described in the Opening Bell (Sun Salutation) in Chapter 5, for building endurance and control in intercourse. The Cobra is similar to the Plank except that the bottom half of the torso is resting on the floor. The third chakra (in the abdomen) is connected to the earth.

Cobra Pose

Time: 30 to 60 seconds

Benefits: Upper body strength, endurance,
and improved sexual functioning

Lying facedown on the floor with hands at sides, inhale and feel the pressure on your hands as you lift your chest along the floor, raising your upper torso, arching your back, and pressing the chest forward while keeping your pelvis and tops of your feet on the floor. Keep your shoulders down, your shoulder blades together, your belly button and lower abdomen on the floor, and your legs outstretched. Keep your chest open and lifted. Push away from the floor as you draw your elbows back. Like a cobra, open your heart center and throat. (See Figure 6.11.) Hold this pose for 30 seconds and then gently lower your body back to the floor.

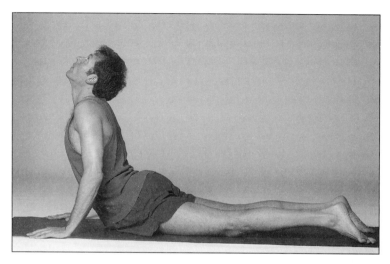

FIGURE 6.11

Kundalini Breathing Exercises

In Kundalini Yoga an image of a great serpent runs from the base of the spine where the serpent rests to the crown of the head, where the lotus flower rests. In Kundalini Yoga you are attempting to bring the Kundalini energy from the lower chakras to the higher ones. This is the basis of the Tantric process. The focus is on the breath, directing the energy upward on the inhalation and downward on the exhalation.

Kundalini Yoga Positions

Maximizing Resources, Deflating a Bloated Bureaucracy, and Timing Acquisitions are especially beneficial for the prostate gland and sexual functioning. (See Chapter 5 for detailed instructions.)

Meditation on Unconditional Love and Lovingkindness

The most rewarding sexual act is to give completely of yourself to your lover without any expectation in return. This meditation's focus is, How can I help? How can I serve? When you are focused on how to please your partner, you take the pressure off yourself to perform and the Universe orchestrates a synchronistic flow of loving energy, allowing you to escape into the timelessness of creation. By giving completely you receive fully, and the experience can only strengthen your love for each other.

Sit on the floor with your legs crossed and back straight (see Chapter 4 for seated postures), or if you're in a chair, sit upright and close

---

Mantras for Meditation

Choose a mantra that has religious or spiritual meaning for you. It will help you concentrate and open your heart chakra.

Hebrew: *To hora he.* (My soul is pure.)

Christian: Amazing grace, open my heart.

Buddhist: *Om mani padme hum.* (The all which is everything blooms in my heart as the lotus flower.)

Yogic/Vedic: *Om shanti in me.* (God and peace in me.)

Moslem: *Salam in me.* (Peace in my heart.)

---

your eyes. Choose one of the following mantras (repetitive sayings) to guide you through this meditation. If your mind wanders, gently bring it back to your mantra. In meditation you learn you are not your thoughts; you are the thinker who has the thoughts. But for now you will quiet those thoughts.

Place your hands on your lower abdomen, and listen as the breath rises and falls. Relax more and more with each breath.

Spend a few minutes following your breath and repeating the mantra until your breathing becomes relaxed. Imagine a ball of white light radiating from your heart throughout your body. End the meditation by coming back in touch with your body, wiggling your fingers and toes, and feeling a warm, tingling sensation through your being.

Tantric Sexual Practices

Through Tantra we can bring spirituality into our sexual experiences. In Tantra, energy is viewed as the source of life. Sexual ecstasy is divine energy. Men can learn to extend arousal before they ejaculate by combining the strength and stamina built up by regular Yoga practice with Kundalini breathing. In particular, you can work toward holding the Plank or Push-up Position (see Opening Bell in Chapter 5) for 30 seconds.

Tantric practices enable us to prolong the sexual experience and heighten the ecstasy. Men can also use the Cobra Pose (Figure 6.11) to delay an orgasm and channel their energy to higher chakras by holding the breath and envisioning the red-orange energies moving upward. Keeping your second and third chakras pressed against your partner will enable you to retain the energy and arousal. Each time you feel that you are going to climax, breathe deeply and tighten your sphincter. Channel the energy to your crown chakra. In this

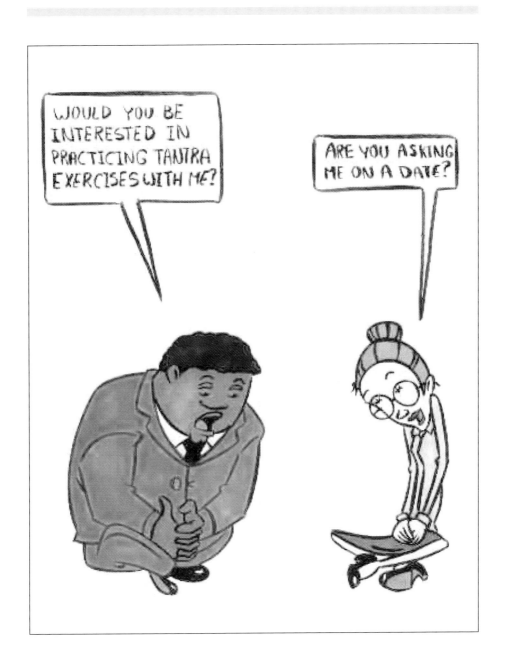

way you can stay aroused for up to forty-five minutes, guaranteeing that your partner will be satisfied and you will achieve a much more powerful sexual experience.

Reiki

Reiki, or energy healing, practiced before intercourse can also heighten the sexual experience. Reiki is an Eastern healing art whereby one partner channels spirit to the other. In this way the receiver can enter a deep state of relaxation similar to that experienced after meditation or deep sleep. Energy levels are restored and you will notice a heightened awareness in all of your senses. This is an opportune time to practice your breathing exercises.

I recommend two simple Reiki exercises to enhance your sexual experience. In the first exercise, stand behind your partner and place your hand on your partner's crown chakra. Hold this position for 2 minutes with the intention of sending loving healing energy. Reverse receiver and giver and repeat.

In the second exercise, face each other with your right hand on your partner's heart chakra and your partner's right hand on your heart chakra. Look into each other's eyes and send lovingkindness.

Sexual Release and Healing for Those Without Partners

Many urologists are convinced that masturbation three or four times per week might help reduce cases of prostate cancer. Diets rich in fat and red meat have elevated men's testosterone levels, and watching sporting events further increases levels of adrenaline and testosterone. Men who are not sexually active are at higher risk for prostate cancer because of the buildup of testosterone and adrenaline in their bodies. So masturbation could help save lives.

The Mind

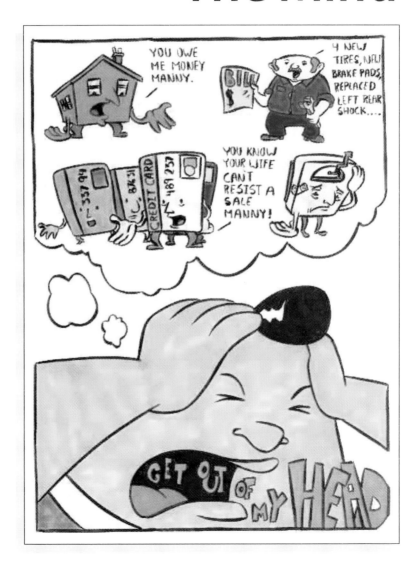

Now that you have worked on Yoga's physical poses, you are ready to learn about the philosophy behind your practice.

Yogic Philosophy

Yoga originated about five thousand years ago in India, but only recently has it reached Western societies. Today more than 18 million Americans regularly practice Yoga. Unfortunately, the focus of many Yoga programs, especially those associated with health clubs, is the body. But Yoga is the union of body, mind, and spirit. The real focus of Yoga is to put you back in your body, in the moment, in touch with your emotions so you can face the normal stresses of life with a firmer footing. Yoga also enables you to communicate, especially to listen, better so you can be more effective in relationships and in the professional world. Yoga is a lifestyle that incorporates the following eight concepts into daily practice through Yoga, meditation, and service to others.

1. OVERCOMING THE CONTROL OF THE EGO

The ego is what keeps us attached to and locked in the prison of our senses. This attachment arises from the survival instinct. As we move our awareness beyond the fight or flight response into heightened states of consciousness, we can more easily identify with the Universe and take a more detached view of events. In this way we can become the masters of our emotions, instead of being their victims. Meditation is a useful way to escape the confines of the ego and see problems from a more enlightened vantage point.

At work this might mean challenging the directives of a superior if you believe you are right. It could mean listening to rather than railing against constructive criticism. Going beyond the confines of your ego means owning your power and staying centered at all times.

It also means being humble, because all beings are equal. If the executive staff gets to know the cleaning and maintenance people on a first-name basis, everyone in the organization is made to feel important. By reducing the hierarchy of command, you empower your human capital and raise the potential of all those in the organization to become cocreators.

At home this may mean giving your children the opportunity to discover their unique talents and not forcing your belief systems on them.

In your relationship with your significant other, this may mean taking a step back from an argument that is repetitive and unproductive. Ultimately this perspective may help you give up controlling others and honor the differences that make your relationships meaningful.

2. MOVING BEYOND DUALISM

The "Western mind" is focused on opposites: good and bad, right and wrong. The need to label everything as one or the other and defend our point of view makes us all warriors. Sometimes we wage war when we should be giving love and compassion. By contrast, Yoga asks us to view things in terms of cause and effect. For example, it might not be inherently evil to modify the genetic makeup of corn so it is resistant to insects; however, monarch butterflies will be affected by this modification, and the biodiversity of the planet will thus be changed.

We spend so much of our energy defending our point of view. If we could just free ourselves of the need to convince everybody of our

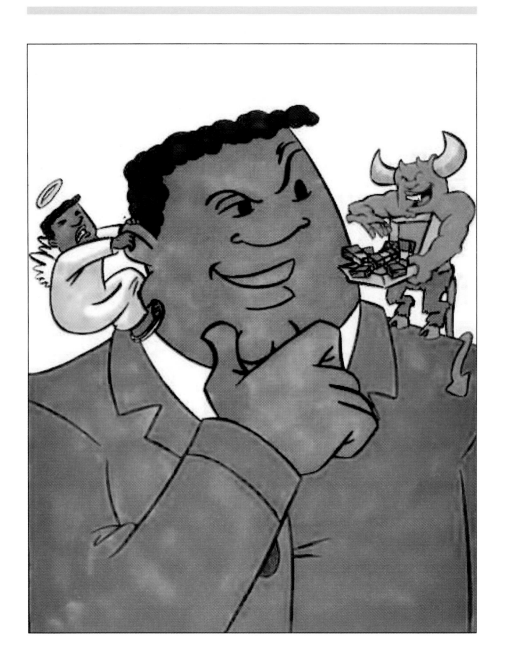

opinion, we could unleash positive energy for more productive pursuits. By understanding cause and effect, we take a detached view of things. Being detached doesn't mean not being concerned. In fact, when you are detached your responses are more compassionate and come from higher states of awareness rather than habitual emotional reactions. By incorporating nonduality into your thought process, you will be able to make more rational decisions without having to wage battles. You will gain a better appreciation for all sides of the story.

3. ASKING, HOW CAN I HELP? HOW CAN I SERVE?

One of the most important concepts in Yoga is service. Ultimately every business organization exists to fulfill a purpose. Encouraging volunteerism among employees is one of the best ways to build an excellent customer service team. If you encourage employees to behave positively in volunteer settings, they are likely to exhibit these same behaviors in the service of your customers. Thus a chain reaction of positive behavior can extend beyond the workplace.

Before you meet with potential clients or customers, try spending some time to focus on lovingkindnes. This practice will help you focus on their needs as opposed to your ego, which is telling you that you must close the deal. By focusing on how you can help and serve, you instantly change the direction of energy from receiving to giving. The pressure is taken off both parties. The key is to focus on giving without the expectation of something in return. You will find that you become a better listener and your potential customers will immediately sense the mutuality of your approach and respond accordingly.

It is very empowering to replace the need to close a transaction with How can I help? How can I serve? You may also find that you are coming up with solutions that will create greater loyalty in the long run. In this way your business relationships will survive ever-shortening product life cycles and, by having opened communication with your customers, you will be able to continue refining your product or service to meet their changing needs.

An example is Mary Kay Cosmetics, a Christian-based company. Their motto is "God first, family second, and company third." The key to their success was to develop a culture where values, especially family, community, and spirit, are respected. The Marriott hotel chain, a Mormon-based company, uses a similar approach to develop excellent customer service skills. With the blurring of the lines between personal life and business, organizations that create a balanced life approach will maximize their human capital and outperform their competitors.

I have founded Yoga for Business, which helps companies train employees and executives to use spiritual practices to improve motivation and customer service and to encourage change.

In our personal lives the focus on How can I help? How can I serve? can be extremely beneficial in sexual relationships, as was discussed in Chapter 6. I suggest using the Lovingkindness Meditation before lovemaking. When you are focused on how you can serve your partner, you will be released from performance anxiety. In addition, changing the focus away from your gratification will paradoxically bring you more gratification because your partner will sense the energy exchange and will feel a heightened arousal. By focusing on how you can serve you will also find yourself slowing down and enjoying the moment.

Service is also key to raising children. Instead of feeling burdened by the demands of your family, you can rejoice and participate in activities with a more positive attitude. The emotion of love is very powerful. Try looking at the world through loving eyes each and every day.

Children need to be taught compassion skills in the same way we teach math or science. To have successful relationships, children need to understand how to give to others. I started a Kid's Care Club in my hometown, where I got children involved in helping out in nursing homes and homeless shelters. I recommend these activities for all children age four and older.

4. UNDERSTANDING KARMA OR PAST ACTIONS

The term *Karma* means "action." Each action you make generates a reaction and a memory associated with that action. The objective of Karma Yoga is to accept your Karma from previous actions so that you don't generate any new Karmic debts. Ultimately we want to transmute our past Karma for the benefit of ourselves and others.

We are bundles of cosmic software, which according to Yogic tradition is called Karma. We are made of the same atoms that existed as a point of light in the beginning of the Universe. So we are walking holograms of creation. Science has shown us that we have mammalian, reptilian, and amphibian structures in our brains. So from a physiological perspective we carry the memories of creation and who we really are. In addition we carry memories of past incarnations, of our race, our species, and so on.

Yoga and meditation help us understand what makes us tick. It is possible to advance to the state where you can use memories instead of allowing memories to use you. When you understand your Karma, you will no longer be a victim of it. You can work on the more important task of transmuting your Karma into your Dharma, which is the reason your soul made this life's journey.

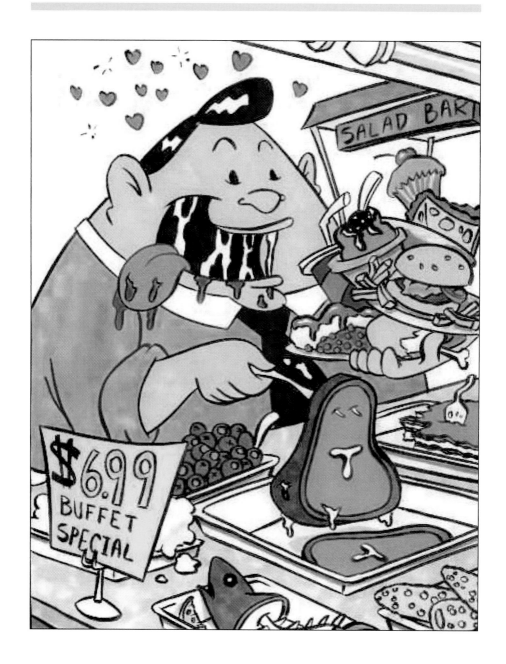

Introduction to Daily Yoga Practice

For example, if in a past incarnation you made your living by selling unhealthy addictive products to others, in your current incarnation you might be a victim of that addiction. To free yourself from that Karma you might start a smoking cessation business. By transmuting your Karma you will not only help yourself but also repay past debts to others. You will alter the flow of energy in the Universe, and the contribution you make will be the most economically beneficial use of your talents. Karma is the hidden force behind many successful business enterprises.

As we progress through various incarnations, we are accompanied by other souls with whom we have shared past Karma. Yoga and meditation help us understand our relationships with family, friends, and co-workers from a broader, more universal perspective and may help us develop compassion for others who are struggling. We don't have to solve everyone's problems, and we certainly do not have to take responsibility for the actions of others. But we can become better listeners and lead by example.

Understanding Karma may mean letting our children make mistakes, even though we want to shelter them from the pain.

By focusing on how you can serve others, you will generate good Karma. An abundance of good Karma will make it easier to accomplish your goals and move toward Dharma. If you can take a painful experience, turn it around, and help others in the process, you gain positive Karma. With meditation you will begin to uncover your Karma and devote attention to living a life of purpose.

5. ENHANCING (SYNCHRONICITY)

The regular practice of meditation will increase and enhance the synchronistic moments of your life. The dictionary defines *synchronicity* as a coincidence of events in which there is simultaneous action that is related. For example, you pick up the phone to call someone and find him or her on the other line.

Synchronicity can be used in many areas of your life: to build a business, form an advisory board, find a strategic partner, or meet your soul mate. Consider that every person you meet offers you an opportunity to learn and grow. By staying alert and in the moment, you can capitalize on opportunities when they arise. Daily Yoga practice will help you to refine these sensibilities.

I have also used synchronicity when on vacation. Vacation is the best time to practice getting comfortable with stepping into the unknown and letting go. The known is our past; there is no growth there. When you go on vacation try to go to different places and seek out adventure. There are newfound friends to be made, different countries to learn about, and interesting places to explore. In a recent trip to the Dominican Republic we dined with new friends, explored waterfalls, journeyed through rain forests, and enjoyed learning about life in that country.

Each day you'll begin to let go of your judgments and expectations and enjoy yourself even more. Yoga will help to open the mind so you can experience the unlimited possibilities in life and find that your desires are fulfilled with less effort.

6. RECOGNIZING HIDDEN MOTIVATIONS AND MEANINGS

Yoga can be extremely powerful in improving the relations within an organization or a family. When practiced in a group, Yoga can help members:

Get in touch with their emotions and empathize with others;

Feel more comfortable with themselves;

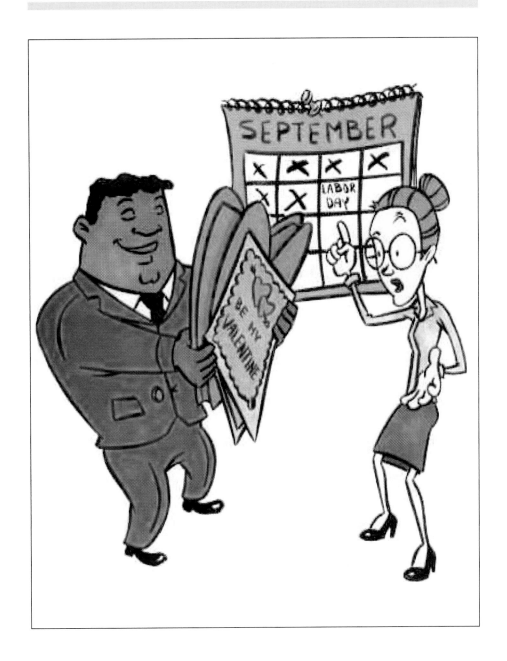

Improve communication both among peer groups and across hierarchical lines;

Create a feeling of belonging to a whole whose sum is greater than its parts, enhancing organizational integration and uniting employees behind common goals.

In the family setting these principles can help us avoid hurt, which can become anger. For example, your parents may be confrontational and grumpy. Perhaps they are in pain, or maybe they are not happy with the way they live their lives. Try to use the Lovingkindness Meditation the next time you are with difficult family members. Smile at them and send them love. Remember that it is not your responsibility to solve their problems. It *is* your responsibility to be compassionate and to send love.

7. FOCUSING ON THE PROCESS

Runners training for a marathon will tell you that they do not focus on the entire task, they take one step at a time. By staying in the moment and focusing on the process, you can become much more effective in accomplishing goals. When you focus only on the outcome you lose spontaneity and the flow of creative energy dries up.

You can practice using the stuff of your daily life as fertile ground for your meditation. The Healthy Living Wellness series includes a number of exercises that help us to eat, walk, drive, and even shop more mindfully. Ultimately all of your actions can become part of the meditative state so that you will be looking at the world through loving eyes. This is what it means to be enlightened.

In business we should consider all problems as potential business models because they represent opportunities for creative thinking.

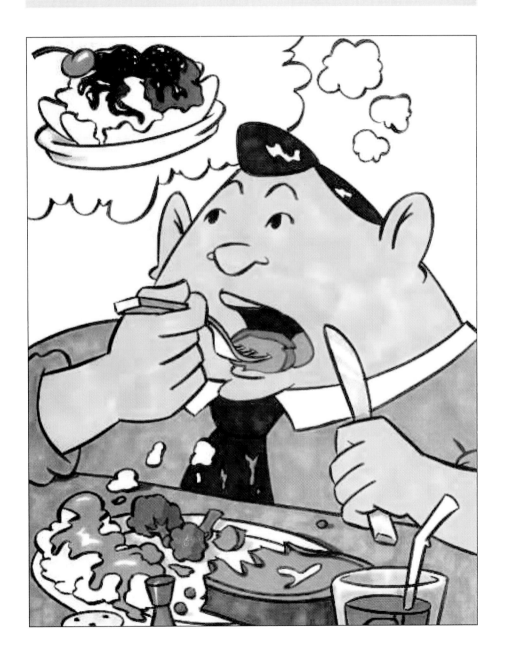

The key is not to force one solution on a problem, which only creates new problems, but to construct several possible solutions. By looking at multiple solutions we're much more likely to reach a positive result. This is the method nature uses to promote evolution and progress. Nature attempts to solve problems by trial and error. All great inventors have had many false starts before they made their discoveries. The key is to suspend judgment and consider false starts not failures but opportunities for further growth. By keeping an open mind we submit ourselves to many learning experiences and opportunities.

8. DISCOVERING DHARMA, OR PURPOSE IN LIFE

Just as every business has a mission or business model, each individual has a special purpose in this life. As Yogis, our most important task is to discover our mission or purpose for this life. Often it is the one thing we can do better than anyone else, and when we are doing this activity we are in a state of timeless awareness, bliss.

For a business organization, helping employees to discover their purpose can be extremely beneficial for productivity and creativity. This approach is tied into the How can I help? How can I serve? concept. If employees truly believe the organization wants to help them grow and develop, they will respond by giving their all back to the company. In addition the company will be more willing to evaluate employees' strengths and facilitate job transfers and retraining. It is a win-win situation for everyone.

On our paths to pursue our Dharma, our spouses or significant others may be helpful, especially if they are open to exploring their own paths. But when spouses or significant others feel threatened because they are resistant to change, they may become obstacles. Although such change can be difficult and painful, the relationships may have to be reevaluated so that we can proceed with our evolution.

It is very important to help our children discover their Dharma. Often we either push our children to pursue our dreams or use fear to get them to choose a "secure occupation." Much of our unhappiness in life stems from being unfulfilled in our jobs. The key to raising happy and healthy adults is to allow children to find their own path and provide guidance when necessary.

Balance

The pose called Firm Footing in a Changing Marketplace in Chapter 5 is a metaphor for a state of mind. In this exercise, try to balance on one foot. If you lose your balance, you can catch yourself with the other foot. You can begin to view your life in this way so you become less resistant. Now switch feet. This exercise if practiced daily will help you to incorporate the belief that you can be flexible to changes in your environment and you will always land on your feet. This exercise may also be useful in balancing left- and right-brain functions and improving mental clarity.

Try to solve problems using all your senses. We all have a bias toward using one of our senses and subjugating the others. We need to bring the rest of our senses into the equation and trust our gut reactions. Use all your assets. Spend time in silence each day. Through meditation and focused concentration we can improve our synchronicity, meet the right people at the right time, be prepared when opportunity presents itself, and find what we are here to do.

If a client of yours was running a business and not fully utilizing its assets, it would probably go out of business. As a proactive adviser you would make sure it leveraged all its assets to achieve its business

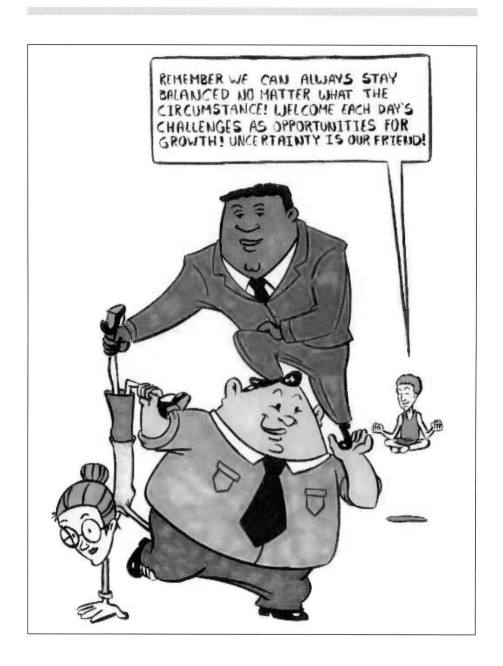

goals. Many of us are not using all our potential; we are running on one brain hemisphere and using only one or two senses. We rarely if ever engage in quiet contemplative thoughts.

It is important to consider all the technologies that will relieve you of mundane chores because the time freed up can be reallocated to creative business building. You will be empowered by upgrading your skills and repositioning yourself for success in the new economy. But above all, imagine how secure you can feel knowing that you are staying ahead of the changing marketplace. By embracing technology you will remain a competitive and vital force in your industry.

BRINGING LOVE INTO THE WORKPLACE

Fear can be a potent motivating force, but over the long term its effects on human capital can be damaging. If all the participants in the marketplace are motivated by fear, the result is the high turnover and stress management problems we are experiencing in today's fast-paced environment. A more long-term solution would be to change the motivation from fear to love. Love-based motivation will create loyalty and purpose, and the energy levels achieved can be sustained.

In your own business you can move away from a fear-based to a love-based motivation by using a Lovingkindness Meditation to motivate employees and improve customer relations. By calling on your higher self, you can also tap into the "cosmic computer" and get information that will be helpful to your customers and employees.

When we connect with employees at this level, the dialogue becomes more meaningful. Employees will recognize our concern and respond with improved performance. Employees then use the same approach to customers, fellow employees, and others. The lovingkindness virus will spread quickly.

The core of our relationships will then be built on compassion, care, trust, and respect. Developing an excellent customer service base requires having all employees focus on How can I help? How can I serve our customers? The best way to begin to inspire this attitude is with top-level executives and managers.

BRING LOVE INTO THE HOME

We are a touch-deprived society. Human beings were designed to live in groups with a great deal of physical interaction, but we have become isolated even though we live together in condensed metropolitan areas.

A recent cross-cultural study counted physical touches between couples. It is no surprise that developed nations are at the bottom of the list. Go to any health club and you will see people paying large sums of money to have some interaction with their trainers.

For those not in committed relationships I strongly recommend having a pet. Studies have shown that interaction with our pets can help us live longer, happier lives. Your pet will also benefit. If you purchase the companion video to this book you will notice that I practice Yoga with my dog Goodboy, a Dalmation. By practicing regularly, Goodboy has become one of the most mellow dogs.

For those in committed relationships time must be made for communicating through touch. Busy couples might have to schedule a date. Massage and gentle stroking are very stimulating and can be excellent methods of foreplay. They are also ways to put the How can I help? How can I serve? principle into operation. Touch is most powerful when you do the Lovingkindness Meditation before and during the massage.

Anyone who has a compromised immune system should consider weekly massage either from a loved one or a paid professional.

CHAPTER
EIGHT
The Spirit

As a species we have suffered 5.9 million years. The first two and a half million years we were oppressed by our environment. Then when we became masters of our world we began to oppress our fellow humans.

Many people ask how we can believe in an intelligent Universe when our history is littered with inequity and strife. When we experience these horrible events we may question the apparent randomness of the Universe. This illusion can be pierced through Yoga and spiritual practice.

Almost every group of people has been a victim of oppression. The Holocaust, in which 12 million souls perished, is a dreadful event in human history. But what if those souls made a supreme sacrifice to raise the level of consciousness of humanity? Did this horrific event raise our awareness of the dangers of hate and violence? Have we evolved into a more peaceful world order as a result of these sacrifices?

After the most recent tragedy at the World Trade Center and the Pentagon and the fighting that has ensued, it may seem that we are taking some steps backward.

Being in a state of elevated consciousness allows us to recognize that the departed souls helped to elevate our consciousness and raise awareness to the hate that certain groups foment. They have protected us against even worse disasters and they continue to protect us from afar.

Love is much more powerful than hate. This has been proved over and over again throughout the ages. The battle against hate can only be won by changing the hearts and belief systems of the people.

A few years ago I was at the Wailing Wall for a Shabbat service. I sat down and began to meditate as as I touched the wall. As a descendant of Abraham and Moses I felt a profound sadness for the suffering of my people. As the commotion began to calm I got into a very deep state and lost all connection to self. The message I got from spirit was that there is no holy place; all place are holy. Spirit cannot be tied to a location in space or a moment in time. It doesn't have these properties.

It is a profoundly tragic cosmic joke to have misinterpreted the nature of the divine in such a way that we destroy in the name of the divine. This is the source of much of our self-inflicted pain and it can be overcome through liberation from limited thinking.

I was later told that, as the night wore on, groups of religious leaders stopped to observe me meditating at the wall. First arrived a group of Greek Orthodox priests, then rabbis and Japanese tourists. When I regained consciousness it was dark and almost two hours had passed. A dear friend told me what had happened. I will always cherish that experience as an awakening for me.

Slavery was yet another crime against humanity that caused much pain and suffering. But is it possible that the millions of souls involved in this barbaric and brutal captivity were sacrificed to create a nation of diversity? Isn't America inspiring in its diversity and tolerance of different ethnic and religious persuasions? While we may not comprehend the methods of the Universe, it's possible these horrible events occurred for higher reasons.

We have all been victims at some point in our lives. The key to leading an enlightened life is to avoid the "victim trap." Feeling victimized is the most crippling form of ignorance because it tells us that we are helpless and insignificant. We have become a nation of victims. Being victims excuses us from responsibility for our actions and gives ammunition to those who are prejudging us. In the most extreme circumstances, victimization can breed hatred and violence toward others, even when the victimization is self-inflicted. The victim trap also retards spiritual evolution and the healing process. Yoga can let us view the victimizing events as spiritual lessons. If you can control your emotions you will recognize these opportunities to grow and evolve. The alternative is experiencing the same Karmic episodes again in your next incarnation.

Forgiveness is another important Yoga concept. It holds the key to unlocking your potential to grow spiritually. Often I end my meditation by praying for people who have hurt me or treated me unfairly. I forgive them and send them love. This is a very freeing and liberating experience. When we forgive others, we empower ourselves. If you can forgive the jerk who cuts you off on the highway, you can avoid the normal reaction of the stress response. In this way you can become a master of your own physiology.

I believe that the forgiving energy we send can have profound effects on other people's behavior. We may still have to defend ourselves against these adversaries, but by letting go of the hate and anger we will be more effective in upholding our values.

For spiritual practice to be effective we need to move away from the melodrama of the daily news. This doesn't mean you should be ignorant about what is going on in the world, but your emotional attachment to it must be diminished. Focus on news sources that offer objective coverage of events. When negativity and sensationalism are used to sell a story, negative Karma is produced. Clouding the mind with disturbing images will also interfere with meditation. Empowering oneself means limiting the power of the media over your life. Only through the introduction of spirit can we have a more loving and compassionate world.

The ultimate purpose of Yoga is to promote spiritual development. Sometimes you have to give your life up in order to save it. The Buddha once said, "This life of ours is as transient as autumn clouds. Watching the birth and death of beings is like watching the movement of a dance. A lifetime is like a flash of lightning in the sky, like a torrent flowing down a steep mountain. We have stopped for a while to love, to share, but this moment is transient, ephemeral. If we share with lightheartedness and love, then this moment will have been worthwhile."

When we can view the movement of our lives from a place of detachment, we can enjoy the process and begin to see the larger picture. Finding your purpose in life and achieving your Dharma should be your ultimate objective. It is, after all, why your spirit has made the journey; there was a lesson to be learned. Through meditation and regular Yoga practice you can begin to understand your Karma and design a program to transmute any Karmic debts. In addition, at a subtle level you will begin to experience your Dharma, and a path will unfold that will lead you toward enlightenment.

To be successful on our path to enlightenment, we will need to understand certain concepts, such as the "space-time illusion," and learn to use tools such as meditation, mudras, and affirmations to overcome limiting belief systems. The following section introduces the tools you will need on your spiritual journey.

Understanding the Space-Time Illusion

We have been deceived by our senses into believing that we live in a material world. For example, there is a whole ecosystem residing under our bedcovers that we don't see. If we did we might not want to go to sleep. Our senses tell us that objects are material, but physicists know they are made mostly of energy.

We are currently witnessing a major evolution in our understanding of life, and science is beginning to confirm what the ancient mystics have been saying for thousands of years. The great physicists now tell us that time may be circular, not linear as we thought. The Universe is a series of expansions and contractions of mind-boggling proportions. Physicists also tell us that we may be in several dimensions at one time. That is, our physical bodies are like the images on a television screen. You are not really material but a projection of energy and information coming from a quantum field. The key is to understand the broadcasting process of your spirit.

Scientists have been studying black holes, extremely large areas where normal laws of physics do not apply. Light cannot escape from these regions, and in them all notions of time and space are turned upside down. It is possible that these unique areas may be windows to other dimensions of reality.

Since we are made of the same stuff as the Universe, the elements of the black holes are inside us. When we go into deep states of transcendence during meditation, we are really entering a familiar dimension that is a natural part of us as much as it is a natural part of the Universe. I think of it as going home.

But what is the darkness, the silence we experience during meditation? I like to think of it as the womb of creation, the unlimited possibilities for the expression of universal intelligence. For example, in music the silence gives the notes their meaning. There are infinite possibilities for the way the notes are arranged. When the sound ends it doesn't die but merely returns to where it came from. Without the silence, the music or tones would have no meaning.

In life, the silence of meditation helps reveal the meaning of our existence. So the most important thing you can do each day is to meditate. Through meditation you will create the music of your life.

Meditation

Meditation is a mental process that involves focusing one's attention to detach one's awareness from the objects of the senses. The meditation can be either objectless or focused. It is recommended that beginners focus on an object.

Here is one of the images Ram Dass uses to describe the essence of the meditative state: Have you ever been walking along the beach when you got lost in the totality of the moment? The feeling of the sand on your feet, the warmth of the sun on your shoulders, the gentle movement of hairs on your arm as a breeze picked up. You weren't thinking, They're looking at me, or concerned about yourself. You had surrendered to the moment, and your every step was gentle and deliberate. Your breathing had also slowed and you were aware of a heightened sense of smell, in fact all your senses were more focused, but you were not being pulled by the senses. This is the beginning of the meditative mind.

Focusing the meditative mind can be based upon a physical experience to begin with. For example, every time I sail my Sunfish I have this experience. When I catch the wind at the right angle and lean my body over the edge of the boat, I become one with the boat and the elements. I am not concerned about how messy my hair looks or the spray of the salt water on my body. My breathing becomes very relaxed and my senses become heightened. For me this is a spiritual experience.

I begin to lose track of where my body ends and the boat begins as the time passes unnoticed. There is a feeling of openness, being unbounded by the normal limitations of space and time. In the middle of the bay I can even get the sensation of the curvature of the earth from the pattern and shapes of the clouds bending on the horizon.

You may not always have the opportunity to get out on a sailboat or be in a special place, but you can take the journey in your mind and experience a mini-vacation right now, where you are.

SAILBOAT MEDITATION

Here is an exercise to get your meditation started. Meditation should preferably be done in the same place at the same time every day. Its reason can be enlightenment for the benefit of yourself and others. The sailboat meditation is presented on the enclosed CD. You may want to read through the material first and then use the CD for regular meditation practice.

Begin seated in an upright position, or sitting cross-legged on the floor (see Chapter 4 for seated postures). Keep your back straight but relaxed, with your chest open and neck free. Correct posture is extremely important to open the movement of energy throughout the body. It is also helpful to use a cushion under your sitting bones to stop your legs from going to sleep. Rest your hands comfortably on your lap with palms open and facing upward. Close your eyes, take an inventory of your body, and relax any areas that are tense. Take a couple of deep belly breaths. Imagine the sounds of the gentle waves as they lap against the boat and the shades of indigo and green in the sails. Your feet are in the hull to support your weight. As you trim the sails, the boat picks up speed and you are sailing off into a brilliant sunset.

If you are distracted by your thoughts, you will drift off course, the sails will fill with air, and your progress will be halted. Come back and focus on the image of the sail, the destination, the purpose. You are the vessel that can maneuver through the water, letting your thoughts drift by like waves, no matter how compelling they are. You are struck by the beauty of the total scene, but you are focused on nothing specific.

As you come ashore you notice an unusual stone glimmering in the water. You pick it up and put it in your pocket. This is your gift from this special place. You follow a trail of tall dune grass glistening in the afternoon sun and settle in a shaded area where soft breezes are whispering through the trees. It is here you will receive your mantra.

In this special place where the ancient Native Americans once watched the strange European vessels arriving, you feel the presence of these wise ones and the gift they are about to bestow upon you. Their gift is to name your boat after a mantra; this way, wherever you are you can sail through your thoughts and stay unattached.

Choose a mantra that has the most meaning for you.

Hebrew: *To hora he* (My soul is pure.)

Buddhist: *Om mani padme hum* (The all is a precious jewel which blooms as the lotus flower in my heart.)

Christian: Amazing grace, open my heart.

Hindu: *Om shanti in me* (God, peace in me.)

Moslem: *Salam in me* (Peace in me.)

I am love.

Body is pure mind is pure spirit is pure.

Repeat your mantra seven times as you follow your breath. With your mantra and your special stone to remind you of this journey, set sail back to your present reality. You may begin to get a sensation of being back in the room, noticing the sounds around you. You may want to wiggle your toes, move your hands, and stretch to bring your body back to a full state of consciousness.

The mantra can be used anytime. You may be walking along a crowded street feeling isolated and unnerved by the panoply of activity vying for your attention, but if you stay with the mantra, you can be quiet inside and continue to view the world with loving eyes. The meditation you just experienced was a guided visualization, which is recommended for beginners to get an appreciation of the meditative state. It is a tool, which can be used until you feel you no longer need it.

Your meditation focus can be on any one of the following:

A bodily sensation (breathing)

A mantra (a repeated sound or phrase that can be used in conjunction with breathing)

A bodily location (such as one of the seven chakras)

A visualization (creative imagination)

A thought (for example, peace or love; this can be combined with the mantra)

An external object, such as a flame or a flower

The breath is my favorite focus because it is the natural rhythm and intelligence of life that courses through your physiology. It may be helpful to wear soft wax earplugs, which heighten the silence and accentuate your breathing. The earplugs can help you block out any distracting noises in your environment. The mantras I just listed are especially effective in opening the heart chakra.

A meditation time of fifteen to twenty-five minutes is recommended. At the end of the meditation you can choose to ask a question about a pressing problem. You may be amazed to find how easy it is to solve problems in this enlightened and detached mode. You can also choose to say a prayer for loved ones and friends that are facing challenges or ask spirit to walk with you in all your steps during the day.

Your ego may come up with many ways to disrupt your meditative practice:

Doubt

Fear

Boredom

Physical discomfort

Plans and to-dos

Negative thoughts

Past hurts

Feelings of superiority

In order to get past these distractions, use either the sailboat image or the following leaf in the stream method (from Ram Dass). When you get caught up in a distracting thought, imagine it is an autumn leaf that has just fallen into the stream and gotten caught on the side. Gently nudge the leaf back into the flowing water, and watch it be carried away. Do not get upset, because your awareness will get caught many times. Through dogged persistence and faith you will eventually arrive at an awareness of your life that is more flexible and flowing.

Many people find that meditation is the most difficult part of Yoga practice, but it is critical. The Universe has existed for billions of years; your life span in this form is only about eighty. The investment of time you make in meditation will assist in your spiritual development beyond the narrow time frame of these living boundaries.

Hand and Eye Mudras

When you look at images of the Buddha you will notice that the hands and eyes are often in different positions. These stylized positions, called mudras, identify specific attitudes or relationships to the Universe. For example, hands together in a prayerful attitude will accentuate peace of mind.

Each mudra corresponds to an energy flow in the body and mind. As in reflexology, where a part of the foot is associated with an organ, mudras can be very powerful in opening channels to certain parts of the mind and body. Some of the mudras are incorporated into different Yoga poses. For example, the prayer mudra, powerful when doing balancing exercises, is used at the beginning of the Opening Bell and Firm Footing in a Changing Environment poses.

There are other mudras suited for meditation as well. For example, the guyan mudra, in which the tip of the thumb touches the index finger, stimulates knowingness and imparts receptivity. It is often used with the lotus position during meditation.

There are also a number of eye mudras that you can practice before beginning your meditation session. These improve learning, attention span, creativity, and memory retrieval. They also help activate the five codes of intelligence, which are sight (visual), sound (auditory), touch (kinesthetic), taste (gustatory), and smell (olfactory), and the sixth sense, intuition. The following is a list of eight eye mudras and their benefits:

Mudra 1: Looking up and to the left, stimulates visual memory

Mudra 2: Looking down and to the left, stimulates auditory memory

Mudra 3: Looking down and to the right, retrieves kinesthetic (touch) memory

Mudra 4: Looking up and to the right, creates new visual expression

Mudra 5: Looking horizontally and to the right, creates new auditory expression

Mudra 6: Looking at the point between your eyes, stimulates the pineal gland, linked to intuition

Mudra 7: Looking at the nose, stimulates olfactory (smell) memory

Mudra 8: Looking at the tongue, stimulates gustatory (taste) memory

Mudras are an important part of Yoga practice. Performing eye mudras about two minutes before meditation will help deepen and strengthen your practice. Medical studies have shown that eye mudras are also excellent tools to induce relaxation and can be used during the day as a relaxation technique.

Daily Affirmations

Practicing daily affirmations is meditation in action, the essence of a spiritual life. The following daily affirmations, to be recited at the end of your meditation, are a combination of the virtues listed by the Yoga master Patanjali in his Yoga Sutra and other Yoga principles.

I will maintain an attitude of lovingkindness to all people and things. (Lovingkindness includes sympathy, compassion, patience, humility, and forgiveness.)

I will always speak the truth.

I will never take what is not mine. (This includes material as well as nonmaterial possessions, for instance, bootlegged music or credit for another's work.)

I will observe devotion and loyalty to family and friends.

I will overcome the trap of greed. (Remember to repeat "Enough is enough" before making a purchasing decision.)

I will never give up on my goals and vision.

I will be patient (There is a time and place for good things to manifest.)

I will stay unattached but in the moment.

I will exercise discipline through daily Yoga practice.

In this chapter we explored the specific methodology developed over thousands of years by the ancient yogis for accessing your spiritual self and living a more rewarding life. I hope this information will be helpful in motivating you to move forward on your inward journey.

CHAPTER
NINE
The Future

We are the product of billions of years of evolution, and it is through us that the Universe is becoming aware of its magnificence. If we choose an enlightened path we will realize that we no longer have to spend all our energy on meeting our basic needs or fighting for survival. Technology is eliminating repetitive tasks and freeing up our time so we may evolve to become cocreators of our Universe. We have the potential to solve every problem and challenge that humankind is facing. With technology we can create a perfect democracy if our citizens empower themselves with knowledge and assume responsibility for decision making.

Yoga can help us to more effectively communicate with people. Our Karma is to bring love into the hearts of every soul on the planet. Spirit is patient and has not limited us from accomplishing this goal by restricting our time to one lifetime. Our progress is built on our past accomplishments.

Yoga can help empower us with the tools to make our lives and our world a better place. Going within is not a retreat but a renewal, an affirmation of life and your contribution to it. All change starts with an individual and radiates outward. I hope this book inspires you to make this world better for yourself and all those around you.

By purchasing this book you have taken a proactive step to improve not only your health but the health of others. If you feel that this book has been helpful to you, please recommend it to a friend.

I wish you abundance in every aspect of your life.

Om Shanti (God and peace.)

Namaste (The Spirit in me honors the spirit in you.)

Appendix
Determining Your Ayurvedic Constitution

The following chart can help you determine your Ayurvedic constitution. In the book, Annie is a Vata, Oscar is a Pitta and Manny a Kapha. You may find that your archetype straddles more than one class, but you will be dominant in one area. Please take the time to fill out the chart indicating with V/P/K in the second column.

Obser-vations	V/P/K	Vata (Air and Space)	Pitta (Fire with Water)	Kapha (Water and Earth)
Body size		Slim	Medium	Large
Body weight		Low	Medium	Overweight
Skin		Thin, dry, cold, rough, dark	Smooth, oily, warm, rosy	Thick, oily, cool, white, pale
Hair		Dry brown, black, knotted, brittle, thin	Straight, oily, blond, grey, red, bald	Thick, curly, oily, wavy, luxuriant, all colors
Teeth		Protruding, big, roomy, thin gums	Medium, soft, tender gums	Healthy, white, strong gums
Nose		Uneven shape, deviated septum	Long pointed, red nose-tip	Short, rounded, button nose
Eyes		Small, sunken, dry, active, black, brown, nervous	Sharp, bright, grey, green, yellow/red, sensitive to light	Big, blue, calm, loving
Nails		Dry, rough, brittle, break easily	Sharp, flexible, pink, lustrous	Thick, oily, smooth, polished
Lips		Dry, cracked, black/brown tinged	Red, inflamed, yellowish	Smooth, oily, pale, whitish
Chin		Thin angular	Tapering	Rounded, double
Cheeks		Wrinkled, sullen	Smooth, flat	Rounded, plump

Obser-vations	V/P/K	Vata (Air and Space)	Pitta (Fire with Water)	Kapha (Water and Earth)
Neck		Thin, tall	Medium	Big, folded
Chest		Flat, sunken	Moderate	Expanded, round
Belly		Thin, flat, sunken	Moderate	Big, potbellied
Hips		Slender, thin	Moderate	Heavy, big
Joints		Cold, cracking	Moderate	Large, lubricated
Appetite		Irregular, scanty	Strong, unbearable	Slow, but steady
Digestion		Irregular, forms gas	Quick, causes burning	Prolonged forms muscus
Taste, healthy preference		Sweet, sour, salty	Sweet, bitter, astringent	Bitter, pungent, astringent
Thirst		Changeable	Surplus	Sparse
Elimination		Constipation	Loose	Thick, oily sluggish
Physical activity		Hyperactive	Moderate	Sedentary
Mental activity		Always active	Moderate	Dull, slow
Emotions		Anxiety, fear, uncertainty	Anger, hate, jealousy, determination	Calm, greedy, attachment
Faith		Variable	Intense, extremist	Consistent, deep mellow
Intellect		Quick but often faulty response	Accurate response	Slow exact
Recollection		Recent good, remote poor	Distinct	Slow and sustained
Dreams		Quick, active, many fearful	Fiery, war, violence	Lakes, snow, romantic
Sleep		Scanty, broken up, sleeplessness	Little, but sound	Deep, prolonged
Speech		Rapid, unclear	Sharp, penetrating	Slow, monotonous
Financial		Very tight with money, concerned about security	Balanced but will spend money on luxuries	May be rich but spends in excess

Reprinted with permission from the *Complete Book of Ayurvedic Home Remedies,* Vasant Lad, Three River Press, 1999.

After finishing the chart, add up the number of marks under vata, pitta and kapha to discover your own balance. Most people will have one archetype predominant, a few will have two archetypes approximately equal and even fewer will have all three archetypes in equal proportion.

PROFILES

The characters in our book series represent the three Ayurvedic archetypes. For each we highlight their mental, behavioral, physical, financial and management traits and specific exercises that relate to their archetypes.

Annie Thracks

Ayurvedic Type: Vata

Mental Indications:
Worry, anxiety
Overactive mind
Impatience
Loss of mental focus
Short attention span
Depression, Psychosis

Behavioral Indications:
Insomnia
Fatigue
Inability to relax
Restlessness
Poor appetite

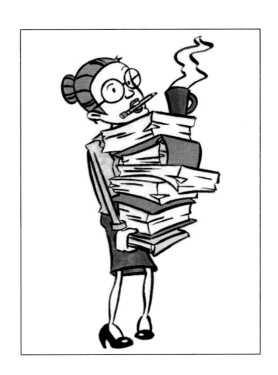

Physical Indications:
Constipation
Dry or Rough Skin
Low Stamina, loss of energy
Intestinal gas
High blood pressure

Financial Profile:
Very critical of financial decision making
Experience anxiety over financial decisions
Very conservative in investments

Management Profile: Obsessive

Exercises to Overcome Obsessive Behavior:
One of the major problems with obsessive employees/managers is the inability to listen. Listening allows the employee/manager to retain focus and will ultimately be more pleasant for the people he or she reports to or depends on.

The Lovingkindness Meditation is especially helpful in improving listening skills. We recommend that you record a meditation in your voice focusing on opening the heart. A mantra such as "How can I help, how can I serve" may be chosen. You might want to listen to this tape on the way to work, or if you are willing to sit down to meditate in a quiet contemplative state.

Oscar Fodder

Ayurvedic Type: Pitta

Mental Indications:
Anger, hostility
Self-criticism
Irritability, impatience
Resentment

Behavioral Indications:
Outbursts of temper
Argumentative stance
Tyrannical behavior
Criticism of others
Intolerance of delays

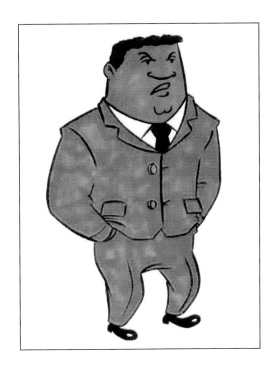

Physical Indications:
Skin inflammations, rashes, acne
Excessive hunger or thirst
Bad breath
Heartburn, acid, ulcers
Sour body odors
Intolerance to heat

Financial Profile:
Career Achiever
Believes that the individual has power over his destiny
Will take risks for potential rewards

Management Profile: Autocratic/Tyrannical

Exercises to Overcome Autocratic/Tyrannical Behavior:
These personality types need to learn to let go of the need for control. Power comes from within and is not based upon the number of people you control.

Successful leaders are able to get the best out of subordinates without using fear by understanding how to motivate the individual. Again the "Lovingkindness Meditation" is very helpful on shifting your focus away form the need to control and toward empowering your staff to perform at their peak.

By focusing on how you can help and serve, you instantly reverse the exchange of energy from receiving to giving. The key is to focus on giving without the expectation of something in return. Have you really ever taken the time to understand your subordinate and the issues of their life?

Manny Problemas

Ayurvedic Type: Kappha

Mental Indications:
Periods of alternating
  creativity and mental
  inertia
Lassitude
Stupor, depression
Overattachment

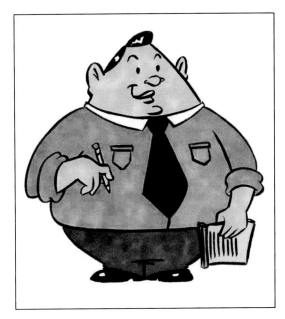

Behavioral Indications:
Procrastination
Inability to accept change
Greed
Oversleeping, drowsiness
Stubbornness
Slow movements
Possessiveness

Physical Indications:
Intolerance of cold/damp
Sinus congestion
Fluid retention, bloating
Chest congestion
Skin pallor
Loose or aching joints
High cholesterol
Allergies, asthma
Diabetes

Financial Profile:
Doesn't believe he has control of financial destiny
Makes financial decisions without much analysis
Feels greater pleasure in spending than saving

Management Profile: Egotistical

Exercises to Overcome Control of the Ego
The ego is what keeps us attached and locked to the prison of our senses. This attachment arises from the survival instinct. As we move our awareness beyond the level of the fight or flight response into heightened states of consciousness, we can more easily identify with the Universe and take a more detached view of events. In this way we can become the masters of our emotions, instead of being a victim of emotions. Meditation and contemplation are useful ways we can escape the confines of our ego, and approach problems from a more enlightened vantage point.

At work, this might mean challenging the directives of a superior if you believe you are right. It could mean listening rather than wailing against constructive criticism that a superior is sharing with you. Going beyond the confines of your ego means owning your own power and staying centered at all times.

It also means being humble, as all beings are equal. If the executive staff gets to know the cleaning and maintenance people on a first name basis, everyone in the organization is made to feel important. By reducing the hierarchy of command in the organization you empower your human capital and raise the potential of the organization to become cocreators.

Now that you have had the opportunity to review Annie, Manny and Oscar's Ayurvedic Archetype you may want to go back to the chart to find out who you most closely identify with.

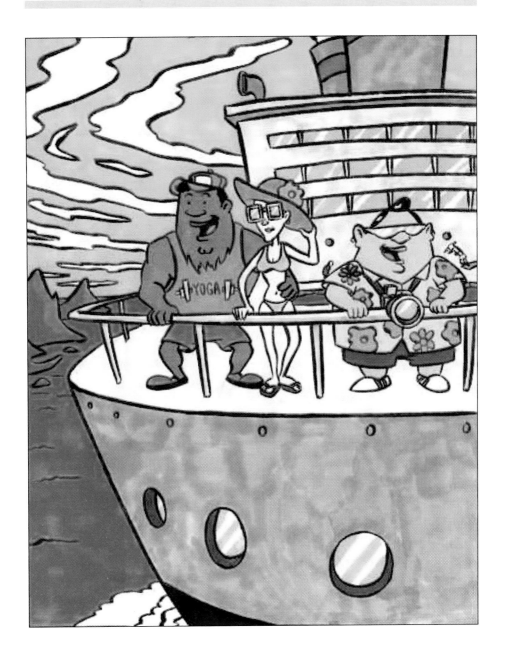

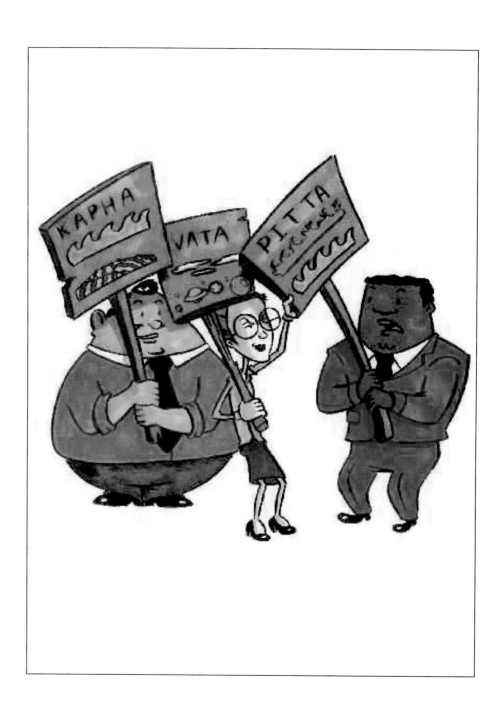

Sound Advice
by Michael DiGirolamo

It is difficult to imagine the impact that sounds have in my life. When I get up in the morning and hear the family of birds that nest in the trees near my house, I react to the rhythmic chirping by assigning it a peaceful sensation, and it sets the tone of my day. If I wake up to a jackhammer in the neighborhood, I react quite differently. I may feel jittery, on edge, or upset, and begin to focus on similar aspects of my life and amplify their significance.

My step is very different when I am at peace, yet energized. I feel somehow lighter. As the day moves on I am exposed to many different sounds that offer themselves for my perception. Most are generated by and for something else, but I sense them and process them. Some are sounds of nature, like wind, rain, wildlife, and surf, which I decide are peaceful, eliciting a response of peace and well-being. Some are made by other people, like jet engines, cars, speech, laughter, air conditioners, footsteps, and alas, music. Some people sounds are unsettling because of sheer volume. Some are contagious like laughter, and tears. All these are presented to us for our decision about them. We make these judgments based on the contexts we have constructed over our lives.

These days, we are exposed to more sounds presented as musical expression, than ever before in our evolution. Up until the advent of recorded sound, if you wanted to hear music, you played it yourself, or attended a concert, or a parade. In tribal society, music is a powerful tool used by a medicine man and is used in ritual and religious ceremonies. Now, it is everywhere. We have devices besides the live performance, which give us musical sounds. Television and radio, are a just a few or the remote devices for music. It is now so commonplace that we don't consciously think about how it is affecting us; it is part of the landscape. But part of us still perceives it and, even if unconsciously, decides what to make of it. The conscious use of music still happens in everyday life, much like it did in tribal days. All religious organizations use music to power their messages. What would a dance club be without the music to set the atmosphere to let go of inhibitions, as in a tribal courting ritual? In an aerobic workout, the rhythm drives the session and energizes the workout. Somebody whose heart was just broken will crave sad love songs to amplify their feelings as a way of understanding what happened, or as a way of deciding how to feel about the event. When I was in high school, we had the state champion wrestling team. At every meet, they would play Locomotive Breath by Jethro Tull as they entered the arena to not only amplify their energy to conquer, but to effectively diminish the power and belief of the opponent. This was a way of making a strong suggestion to a deep part of the opposition's psyche that they would lose. Music is used in a similar way to march people to war. Musical rhythm entrainment is a powerful tool to unify, even if it is about unifying an army.

Carl Jung believed that music had enormous power that was not yet understood by modern man. He argued that music effects the realm of the collective unconscious, the common consciousness of humans. Many in industry use this avenue of communication with the masses to consolidate power, and for monetary gain. They follow the musical formulas discovered by past musicians that have more or less elicited a uniform response among us. Thus manipulating the deep archetypal material in us that Jung described.

Regardless of that behavior, it is still ultimately up to us to make the decision about how we perceive the sounds we hear. We must become more conscious of how these sounds affect us throughout our daily lives, and how we use this vast and available resource ourselves. Learn more about the effects of sound and the perception of music. Choose your CDs carefully. Pay attention to the music you hear on TV. It is in a supporting role, but try just for a moment to imagine a commercial or a movie without any music. Better yet, watch your favorite show or movie, with the sound level off. These exercises will you some idea of the scope of music in your life, especially if you haven't thought about it much.

Vibration does not even have to make a "sound" in order for us to "hear." There has been research done with new imaging technology, indicating that sounds out of our range of audible hearing still stimulate deep centers of brain activity. Those without hearing still hear on some level, perceiving and processing not only these super high and low vibrations, but the subtle vibration of thought. Beethoven was able to express some of his most profound musical feelings without the ability to hear the sounds outside his own mind. The sound of his music has affected generations.

You can use the power of sound yourself, just like others use it on you without you really realizing it. Be more conscious of sound. Music therapists use music as a vehicle for healing because it's perceptions reside so deep that it affords different levels of communication throughout different stages of human life. Music helps people remember, and express things that are buried in our consciousness. It can break down the walls of separation between us, but it can also do the opposite. So be aware of this force that moves the very air we are immersed in, from the little sounds of thought, to the sounds of everyday life, to the way and the reasons why, we organize atmospheric disturbances into music. This knowledge is a most useful tool in self-discovery and healing.

I hope you enjoy the music I have composed on the accompanying CD.

Michael DiGirolamo

Art Therapy
by Robert Bandel

From my own experience I have discovered that sketching or doodling seems to have a relaxing and rejuvenating power to it. I don't know the theories behind it but I know that it works for me. Even if I have been drawing all day long on a commissioned illustration project I get great enjoyment by putting the work aside and sketching some nonsense on a piece of scrap paper. However the sketching should not be taken too seriously. Just let whatever ideas pop into your head flow from the pen or pencil. This will help you relax, burn off a bit of tension and gain back some creative juices you may have lost from concentrating too hard on your work. And you don't have to have art training to be able to doodle. We were all in the same art classes as kids. It's just that some of us got more serious than others in our career choices. But I guarantee the most stuffed shirt corporate exec could come up with a pretty good dog sketch if we forced him to do it. And we might all have a good laugh about it too, which is another stress reliever. I love seeing the sketches that people who claim they can't draw come up with when forced to.

Sketching has been my savior at times. During the summer my girlfriend will drag me to street fairs. It's nice to get out and walk around but I don't care much for the useless junk that most vendors are peddling. So instead of getting all tired, bored and annoyed I bring a sketchbook and draw all the other people throwing away their hard earned money on bottles with colored sand or yet another lawn orna-ment. Having a sketchbook helps if you have to wait in line or some other similarly annoying, unavoidable activity like it. I have had many hours during these waits, of gut busting laughter as my girlfriend and I push the little sketchpad back and forth, and make new additions to it. She is a teacher and not a professional artist but I love the wacky stuff she comes up with.

Another potential stress reliever is to go and see some good art or a decent movie every so often. Subconsciously we are affected by colors, angles and shapes, which can alter our moods. Viewing well-organized and arranged art can be soothing to the sight and the soul, and heal the damage caused by precariously placed shapes and colors of our world today.

The healthcare industry is beginning to understand the importance of the visual aesthetics in the healing process. In a recent article in the *Wall Street Journal,* patients gave themselves 45% less self-administered pain medication after the hospital was redesigned with softer colors like pastel greens and blues and warmer indirect lighting.

Various scientific studies show that exposure to nature reduces stress and speeds healing. When we are unable to bring nature into our environment the next best thing is art and color therapy. The Ancient Yogis understood that color is associated with various energy centers of the body. They developed a system to relate the colors to proven physiological effects.

Black: self-confidence, power, strength (7th chakra)

White: clarity, mental focus (7th chakra)

Violet/Pink: suppresses appetite, provides a peaceful environment, good for migraines (6th chakra)

Blue: calming, lowers blood pressure, decreases respiration (5th chakra)

Green: soothing, relaxing mentally as well as physically, helps those suffering from depression, anxiety, nervousness (4th chakra)

Yellow: energizes, relieves depression, improves memory, stimulates appetite (3rd chakra)

Orange: energizes, stimulates appetite and digestive system (2nd chakra)

Red: stimulates brain wave activity, increases heart rate, respirations and blood pressure, excites sexual glands (1st chakra)

Modern science has begun to confirm what the Yogic philosophers had discovered. Attached to the brain are pineal glands, which control the daily rhythm of life. When light enters the eyes (or the skin) it travels neurological pathways to these pineal glands. Different colors give off different wavelength frequencies and these frequencies have different effects on physical and psychological functioning.

Color therapy can either be practiced by having light bounce off an object or by the use of colored light.

I hope you will start to honor your inner artist and creator, and find time to connect with nature either through direct experience or through the art you bring into your home. I am confident that these tools will help you to live a healthier and more fulfilling life.

Robert Bandel
Artist, illustrator, cartoonist, and art therapist

Humor Therapy

Therapeutic Benefits of Laughter

Dr. Lee Berk and fellow researcher Dr. Stanley Tan of Loma Linda University in California have been studying the effects of laughter on the immune system. To date their published studies have shown that laughing lowers blood pressure, reduces stress hormones, increases muscle flexion, and boosts immune function by raising levels of infection-fighting T-cells, disease-fighting proteins called Gamma-interferon and B-cells, which produce disease-destroying antibodies. Laughter also triggers the release of endorphins, the body's natural painkillers, and produces a general sense of well-being.

Following is a summary of his research, taken from an interview published in the September/October 1996 issue of the *Humor and Health Journal*.

LAUGHTER ACTIVATES THE IMMUNE SYSTEM

In Berk's study, the physiological response produced by belly laughter was opposite of what is seen in classical stress, supporting the conclusion that mirthful laughter is a eustress state—a state that produces healthy or positive emotions.

Research results indicate that, after exposure to humor, there is a general increase in activity within the immune system, including:

- An increase in the number and activity level of natural killer cells that attack viral infected cells and some types of cancer and tumor cells.
- An increase in activated T cells (T lymphocytes). There are many T cells that await activation. Laughter appears to tell the immune system to "turn it up a notch."
- An increase in the antibody IgA (immunoglobulin A), which fights upper respiratory tract insults and infections.
- An increase in gamma interferon, which tells various components of the immune system to "turn on."
- An increase in IgB, the immunoglobulin produced in the greatest quantity in body, as well as an increase in Complement 3, which helps antibodies to pierce dysfunctional or infected cells. The increase in both substances was not only present while subjects watched a humor video; there also was a lingering effect that continued to show increased levels the next day.

LAUGHTER DECREASES "STRESS" HORMONES

The results of the study also supported research indicating a general decrease in stress hormones that constrict blood vessels and suppress immune activity. These were shown to decrease in the study group exposed to humor.

For example, levels of epinephrine were lower in the group both in anticipation of humor and after exposure to humor. Epinephrine levels remained down throughout the experiment.

In addition, dopamine levels (as measured by dopac) were also decreased. Dopamine is involved in the "fight or flight response" and is associated with elevated blood pressure.

Laughing is aerobic, providing a workout for the diaphragm and increasing the body's ability to use oxygen.

Laughter brings in positive emotions that can enhance—not re-place—conventional treatments. Hence it is another tool available to help fight the disease.

Experts believe that, when used as an adjunct to conventional care, laughter can reduce pain and aid the healing process. For one thing, laughter offers a powerful distraction from pain.

In a study published in the *Journal of Holistic Nursing,* patients were told one-liners after surgery and before painful medication was admin-istered. Those exposed to humor perceived less pain when compared to patients who didn't get a dose of humor as part of their therapy.

Perhaps the biggest benefit of laughter is that it is free and has no known negative side effects.

So, here is a summary of how humor contributes to physical health. More details can be found in the article "Humor and Health," con-tributed by Paul McGhee.

Muscle Relaxation Belly laugh results in muscle relaxation. While you laugh, the muscles that do not participate in the belly laugh, re-lax. After you finish laughing those muscles involved in the laughter start to relax. So, the action takes place in two stages.

Reduction of Stress Hormones Laughter reduces at least four of the neuroendocrine hormones associated with stress response. These are epinephrine, cortisol, dopac, and growth hormone.

Immune System Enhancement Clinical studies have shown that humor strengthens the immune system.

Pain Reduction Humor allows a person to "forget" about pains such as aches, arthritis, etc.

Cardiac Exercise A belly laugh is equivalent to "an internal jog-ging." Laughter can provide good cardiac conditioning especially for those who are unable to perform physical exercises.

Blood Pressure Women seem to benefit more than men in preventing hypertension.

Respiration Frequent belly laughter empties your lungs of more air than it takes in resulting in a cleansing effect—similar to deep breathing. Especially beneficial for patient's who are suffering from emphysema and other respiratory ailments.

Pet Therapy

Research has shown that heart attack victims who have pets live longer. Even watching a tank full of tropical fish may lower blood pressure, at least temporarily. A study of 92 patients hospitalized in coronary care units for angina or heart attack found that those who owned pets were more likely to be alive a year later than those who did not. The study found that only 6 percent of patients who owned pets died within one year compared with 28 percent of those who did not own pets.

The therapeutic use of pets as companions has gained increasing attention in recent years for a wide variety of patients—people with AIDS or cancer, the elderly, and the mentally ill. Unlike people, with whom our interactions may be quite complex and unpredictable, animals provide a constant source of comfort and focus for attention. Animals bring out our nurturing instinct. They also make us feel safe and unconditionally accepted. We can just be ourselves around our pets.

Research has shown that pet ownership can:

- **Reduce stress-induced symptoms**

  In a study people undergoing oral surgery spent a few minutes watching tropical fish in an aquarium. The relaxation level was measured by their blood pressure, muscle tension, and behavior. It was found that the subjects who watched the fish were much more relaxed than those who did not watch the fish

Reprinted with permission of Holisticonline.com

prior to the surgery. People who watched the fish were as calm as another group that had been hypnotized before the surgery. Other researchers have found that:

—Petting a dog has been shown to lower blood pressure.
—Bringing a pet into a nursing home or hospital can boost peoples' moods and enhance their social interaction.

• **Require less medical care**

A study conducted at UCLA found that dog owners required much less medical care for stress-induced aches and pains than non-dog owners.

• **Add years to your life**

In a study conducted at City Hospital in New York, it was found that heart patients who owned the pets were significantly more likely to be alive a year after they were discharged from the hospital than those who didn't own pets. The presence of a pet was found to give higher boost to the survival rate than having a spouse or friends.

We should point out in this connection that pets can be a source of stress to some people. They may worry who will take care of their pets when they die. In most cases, however, the need to take care of the pets give a reason for living to many terminally ill patients, prolonging their life span.

What Type of Pet?

It is surprising that it does not matter what the pet is to get the therapeutic benefit. It could be a dog, a cat, parakeet, a gold fish, or anything else. The only thing that matters is that the animal is of interest to you.

However, it is important that the pet you have selected fit your temperament, living space, and lifestyle. Otherwise it will be additional source of stress. So, look over the pet and see whether the chemistry is compatible before you decide to adopt one.

How?

It is possible that people who own pets may have different personality traits than those who do not. Research has found that complex, varied, and interesting daily activity is the strongest social predictor of longevity. Pet ownership may affect people physiologically through the soothing and relaxing effect of touch. And speechless communication with a pet, or simply watching a cat or fish, may produce a relaxation response with little demand on the patient.

Pet owners often feel needed and responsible, which may stimulate the survival incentive. They feel they need to survive to take care of their pets. (Many cancer patients with pets have lived longer because they felt that their pets need them!) Stroking a dog, watching a kitten tumble, or observing the hypnotic explorations of fish can be an antidote to a foul mood or a frazzling day.

Pets such as dogs and cats provide unconditional, nonjudgmental love and affection. And pets can shift our narrow focus beyond ourselves, helping us to feel connected to a larger world.

Selected General References

Anantharaman, V., and Sarada Subrahmanyam. Physiological benefits in hatha yoga training. *The Yoga Review,* 3(1):9-24.

Arpita. Physiological and psychological effects of Hatha yoga: A review of the literature. *The Journal of The International Association of Yoga Therapists,* 1990, 1(I&II):1-28.

Bhole, M. V. Some neuro-physiological correlates of yogasanas. *Yoga-Mimamsa,* April 1977, 19(1):53-61.

Cole, Roger. Physiology of yoga. *Iyengar Yoga Institute Review,* Oct 1985.

Corby, J. C., W. T. Roth, V. P. Zarcone, Jr., and B. S. Kopell. Psychophysiological correlates of the practice of Tantric Yoga meditation. *Archives of General Psychiatry, May 1978, 35(5):571-577.*

Davidson, Julian M. The physiology of meditation and mystical states of consciousness. Perspectives in Biology and Medicine, Spring 1976, 19:345-379.

Delmonte, M. M. Physiological concomitants of meditation practice. *International Journal of Psychosomatics, 1984, 31(4):23-36.*

_____. *Physiological responses during meditation and rest. Biofeedback Self Regulation, Jan 1984, 9(2):181-200.*

_____. *Biochemical indices associated with meditation practice: A literature review. Neuroscience and Biobehavioral Reviews, Winter 1985, 9(4):557-561.*

Dostaleck, C. Physiological bases of yoga techniques in the prevention of diseases. CIANS-ISBM Satellite Conference Symposium, Hanover, Germany, 1992: Lifestyle changes in the prevention and treatment of disease. Homeostasis in Health and Disease, 1994, 35(4-5):205-208.

Ebert, Dietrich. Yoga from the point of view of psychophysiology. *Yoga-Mimamsa,* 28(4):10-21.

Elson, Barry D., Peter Hauri, and David Cunis. Physiological changes in yoga meditation. *Psychophysiology,* January 1977, 14:52-57.

Engel, K. *Meditation, Vol. 2: Empirical Research and Theory.* Frankfurt, Germany: Peter Lang, 1997.

Funderburk, James. *Science Studies Yoga: A Review of Physiological Data*. Honesdale, Penn.: Himalayan International Institute, 1977.

Gopal, K. S., O. P. Bhatnagar, N. Subramanian, and S. D. Nishith. *Indian Journal of Physiology and Pharmacy*, 1973, 17(3):273-276.

Jevning, R., R. K. Wallace, and M. Beidebach. The physiology of meditation: A review. A wakeful hypometabolic integrated response. *Neuroscience and Biobehavioral Reviews, Fall 1992, 16(3):415-424.*

King, Roy, M.D., and Ann Brownstone. Neurophysiology of Yoga meditation. International Journal of Yoga Therapy, 1999, 9:9-17.

Kuvalayananda, Swami. Some physiological aspects of meditative poses. *Yoga-Mimamsa*, 1928, 3(3):245-250.

_____. Physiology of pranayama. *Kalyana-Kalpataru,* 1940, 7(1):219-228.

Majmundar, Matra. *Physiology of Yoga Therapeutics* (working title). Forthcoming.

Malathi, A., Neela Patil, Nilesh Shah, A. Damodaran, and S. K. Marathe. Promotive, prophylactic benefits of yogic practices in middle-aged women. *International Journal of Yoga Therapy*, forthcoming 2001, no. 11.

Motoyama, Hiroshi. *A Psychophysiological Study of Yoga*. Tokyo: Institute for Religious Psychology, 1976.

Murphy, M., and S. Donovan. The Physiological and Psychological Effects of Meditation: A Review of Contemporary Research with a Comprehensive Bibliography 1931-1996. 2d ed. Sausalito, Calif.: The Institute of Noetic Sciences, 1997.

Pero, G., and G. Spoto. Study on the anatomy of yoga asana and their neurological effect: A comparative study. *Yoga-Mimamsa,* 1985, 24(3):17-18.

Roney-Dougal, S. M. On a possible psychophysiology of the yogic chakra system. *Journal of Indian Psychology,* Jul 1999, 17(2).

Sahu, R. J., and M. V. Bhole. Effect of 3 weeks yogic training programme on psychomotor performance. *Yoga-Mimamsa,* 1983, 22(1&2):59-62.

Santha, Joseph, K. Shridharan, S. K. B. Patil, M. L. Kumaria, W. Selvamurthy, and H. S. Nayar. Neurohumoral and metabolic changes consequent to yogic exercises. *Indian Journal of Medical Research,* 1981, 74:120-124.

_____, K. Shridharan, S. K. B. Patil, M. L. Kumaria, W. Selvamurthy, N. T. Joseph, and H. S. Nayar. Study of some physiological and biochemical parameters in subjects undergoing yogic training. *Indian Journal of Medical Research,* July 1981, 74:120-124.

Schell, F. J., B. Allolio, and O. W. Schonecke. Physiological and psychological effects of Hatha-Yoga exercise in healthy women. *International Journal of Psychosomatics,* 1994, 41(1-4):46-52.

Selvamurthy, W., H. S. Nayar, N. T. Joseph, and S. Joseph. Physiological effects of yogic practices. *NIMHANS (National Institute of Mental Health and Neuro Sciences of India) Journal* January, 1983, 1(1):71-79.

Singh, R. H., R. M. Shettiwar, and K. N. Udupa. Physiological and therapeutic studies on yoga. *The Yoga Review,* 1982, 2(4):185-209.

_____, and K. N. Udupa. Psychobiological studies on some hatha-yogic practices. *Quarterly Journal of Surgical Sciences,* 1977, 13(3-4):290-293.

Udupa, K. N., R. H. Singh, and R. M. Shettiwar. Studies on physiological, endocrine and metabolic responses to the practice of 'yoga' in young normal volunteers. *Journal of Research in. Indian Medicine,* 1971, 6(3):345-353.

_____. Studies on physiological and metabolic response to the practice of yoga in young normal volunteers. *Journal of Research in Indian Medicine,* 1972, 6(3):345-353.

_____. Physiological and biochemical changes following the practice of some yogic and non-yogic exercises. *Journal of Research in. Indian Medicine,* 1975, 10(2):91-93.

_____. Physiological and biochemical studies on the effect of yoga and certain other exercises. *Indian Journal of Medical Research,* 1975, 63(4):620-625.

_____. A comparative study on the effect of some individual yogic practices in normal persons. *Indian Journal of Medical Research,* 1975, 63(8):1960-1971.

_____, R. H. Singh, and R. A. Yadav. Certain studies on psychological and biochemical responses to the practice of hatha yoga in young normal volunteers. *Indian Journal of Medical Research,* 1973, 61(2):231-244.

Wallace, Robert, and H. Benson. The physiology of meditation. *Scientific American,* February 1972, 226:84-90.

Wenger, M. A., and B. K. Bagchi. Studies of autonomic functions in practitioners of Yoga in India. *Behavioral Science,* 1961, 6:312-323.

West, Michael A. Physiological effects of meditation: A longitudinal study. *British Journal of Social and Clinical Psychology,* June 1979, 18:219-226.

Woolfolk, Robert L. Psychophysiological correlates of meditation. *Archives of General Psychiatry,* Oct 1975, 32:1326-1333.

For additional references, see the extensive bibliography "Psychophysiological Effects" at the IAYT website, *www.iayt.org/biblio.asp.*

To view abstracts in the Medline database for some of the cited articles, go to *http://www.ncbi.nlm.nih.gov/pubmed* and in the search box enter the complete title of the article. If this generates too many hits or no hits, try entering the names of the article's authors using the following format: Delmonte MM (no comma, no periods following the initials, and no space between the initials; if there is more than one author, separate the names by comma, e.g.: Corby JC, Roth WT, etc.; capitalization is not required).

Healthcare Statistics: William M. Mercer, Inc; Milliman & Robertson Inc; Health Affairs; Census Bureau, Harris Poll; Henry J. Kaiser Family Foundation/Harvard School of Public Health